Prevent Denials
and
Win Appeals

The Hospital Case Manager's Guide to Revenue Integrity

Paul Arias, RN, BSN, MIS

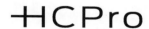

Prevent Denials and Win Appeals: The Hospital Case Manager's Guide to Revenue Integrity is published by HCPro, Inc.

ISBN 978-1-60146-641-9

Paul Arias, RN, BSN, MIS, Author
Janet Morris, Senior Managing Editor
Ilene MacDonald, Executive Editor
Lauren McLeod, Group Publisher
Janell Lukac, Graphic Artist

Leah Jenness, Copyeditor
Karin Holmes, Proofreader
Matt Sharpe, Production Supervisor
Susan Darbyshire, Art Director
Jean St. Pierre, Director of Operations

Advice given is general. Readers should consult professional counsel for specific legal, ethical, or clinical questions.

Arrangements can be made for quantity discounts. For more information, contact:

HCPro, Inc.
P.O. Box 1168
Marblehead, MA 01945
Telephone: 800/650-6787 or 781/639-1872
Fax: 781/639-2982
E-mail: *customerservice@hcpro.com*

Visit HCPro at its World Wide Web sites:
www.hcpro.com and *www.hcmarketplace.com*

9/2009
21710

Contents

About the Author

Paul Arias, RN, BSN, MIS, is the senior director of case management at Inova Fairfax Hospital in Falls Church, VA. He was most recently the director of care coordination at Crouse Hospital in Syracuse, NY, which maintained a denial rate of less than 1% and a 72% reversal rate under his leadership.

In more than 14 years as a nurse, Arias has been primarily in leadership roles, including ED assistant manager, critical care director, and chief executive nurse/director of patient care services. He was a copresenter for HCPro's audio conference "Prevent Denials through Case Management."

Introduction

The purpose of this book is to provide you with information that will lead to a successful implementation of a denial prevention and recuperation program. For years, hospitals have been held liable for a loss of payment because of a lack of medical necessity, demonstrating why a patient needed an admission to an acute level of care. Hospitals have struggled to devise programs to ensure payment, and most efforts have been concentrated on the back end; however, denial prevention begins at the point of entry. As you read through this book, envision the program from the point the patient enters the facility all the way to the payment from the insurance carrier. Many of the topics discussed are tried-and-true methodologies that have led to successful outcomes as the author implemented or assisted others in implementing the strategies outlined herein.

History of Medical Necessity

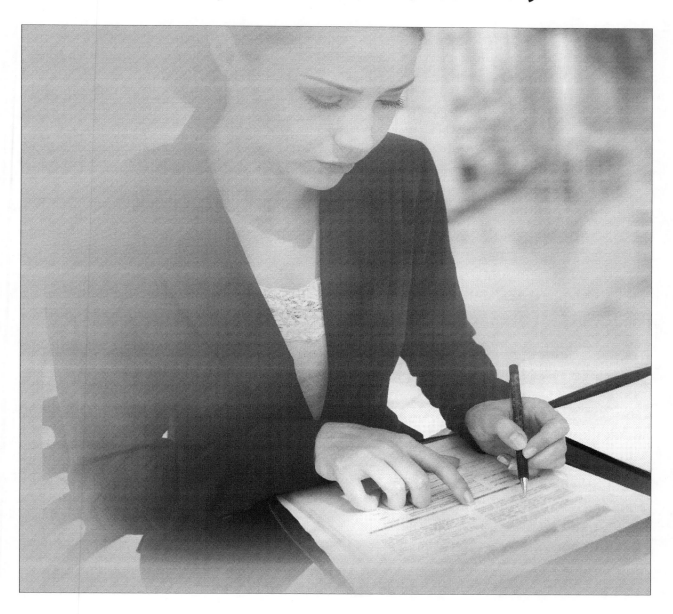

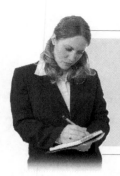

History of Medical Necessity

Medical Necessity Overview

Medical necessity is used in today's healthcare environment to dictate and drive the cost of care so that it is spread as evenly as possible for all beneficiaries. By dividing the cost of care in an even distribution pattern based on medical necessity, insurance companies maintain that they can better serve their members and have sufficient funds to meet the demands of care. From a denial management perspective, medical necessity is one of the most important elements to grasp to be successful in capturing reimbursement for medical services. Denial prevention and money recuperation starts with understanding the importance of a medically necessary admission and continued stay and the documentation that is required to be in the medical record to ensure timely and appropriate payment.

LEARNING OBJECTIVES

At the end of this chapter, the reader should be able to:

✔ Define the basis of medical necessity and its history

✔ Explore how Medicare defines medical necessity

✔ Explain how the case management function fits within the prevention of denials

✔ Briefly review the role of the emergency department case manager in the preemptive prevention of denials

✔ Relate the evolution of evidence-based medical criteria

The Creation of Medical Necessity

The conundrum of medical necessity is how it is defined. To better understand the definition, we must first look at its creation.

During the 1940s, medical insurance plans became a part of the American healthcare system, and medical necessity became an inherent part of the system in order to provide cost savings and spread the ability to provide care for many. The determination of the necessity of care was still relegated to the judgment of the treating physician. The Social Security Act of 1965 established Medicare and Medicaid, and in 1966, Medicare was fully implemented. To control costs, certain mandates were enacted, and by 1972 it was required that each admission to an acute care hospital be reviewed for medical necessity. Under the

Medicare and Medicaid program, the judgment of the physician was placed under scrutiny. Although the program's admitting criteria still observed the physician's judgment as being paramount in the ability to admit a patient, there was a need to look at how admission decisions were made across physician practices. Oversight of the program included a mandate that payment would be made only for appropriate and medically necessary care.

Defining Medical Necessity

Medical necessity was established by Medicare as a means to provide cost-effective care and prevent the treating physician from indiscriminately requesting admission or continued stay. The use of professional services and the need for diagnostic tests also came under scrutiny. The Social Security Amendment contained the provision that "health services ordered for government patients are provided economically and only when, and to the extent, medically necessary" (Blanchard, 2004, p. 601). The problem with that provision was that no true definition of medical necessity was provided. The interpretation held by many was that the government wanted to ensure that physicians provided care "in the context of the shortest, least expensive or least intense in terms of level of treatment of care or service provided" (Blanchard, 2004, p. 601).

Concurrently in the 1970s, private insurance companies began to require that physicians justify their care decisions. This change in practice by the insurance companies led Medicare to begin to issue coverage determinations and start a list of noncovered services. Also thrown into the fray were the Medicaid programs in each state. Some of their definitions included language such as "accepted medical practice or community standards of care; not for the convenience of the patient or provider; not experimental or investigational; and appropriate and effective" (Bergthold, 1995, 180).

The Supreme Court joined in the discussion in 1977 in the case of *Beal v Doe* (U.S. 438, 444), stating that medical necessity within Medicaid programs, known as Title XIX, "conferred broad discretion on the states to adopt standards for determining the extent of medical assistance." The court further stated that "nothing in the language of Title XIX requires a participating state to fund every medical procedure falling within the delineated categories of medical care. Each state is given broad discretion to determine the extent of medical assistance that is 'reasonable' and 'consistent with the objectives.' " The court also stated that "the Social Security Act does not require participating states to fund every medical procedure falling within delineated categories of medical need, but each state is given broad discretion to determine extent of medical assistance that is reasonable and consistent with objectives of the Act, and, although serious questions might be presented if state Medicaid plans did not cover necessary medical treatment, it is not inconsistent with the Act's goals to refuse to fund unnecessary, though perhaps desirable, medical services." Again there was a failure to describe or determine medical necessity.

In 1980, in the case of *Pinneke v Preisser* (623 F 2d 546, 550), the 8th Circuit Court of Appeals recognized that "the decision of whether or not certain treatment or a particular type of treatment is medically necessary rests with the individual recipient's physician and not with clerical personnel or government officials."

In 1998, the AMA released the following definition of medical necessity:

> *Healthcare services or products that a prudent physician would provide to a patient for the purpose of preventing, diagnosing, or treating an illness, injury, disease, or its symptoms in a manner that is: (a) in accordance with generally accepted standards of medical practice; (b) clinically appropriate in terms of type, frequency, extent, site and duration; and (c) not primarily ... for the convenience of the patient, treating physician, or other healthcare provider (AMA Policy H-320.953, 1998).*

Most healthcare plans followed suit and provided similar definitions that included provisions to:

- *Prevent the onset or worsening of an illness, condition, or disability*

- *Provide palliative, curative, or restorative treatment for physical and/or mental health conditions*

- *Establish a diagnosis*

- *Assist the individual to achieve or maintain maximum functional capacity in performing daily activities, taking into account both the functional capacity of the individual and those functional capacities that are appropriate for individuals of the same age (Blanchard, 2004, p. 602)*

As recently as the Clinton administration, a better definition of medical necessity was debated in Congress, but no consensus was reached. Language in the debate included "effective," "beneficial," and "judicious." Each of these terms carries its own interpretation that can be ambiguous and can lead to further confusion. What is "beneficial" and to whom is the benefit applied? What about "judicious"? How would that apply to the beneficiary, versus what the plan determines to be judicious? Because there were many stakeholders, each with their own needs and agenda, including the different political parties, the drive to create a national health plan that included a working definition of medical necessity died a slow death in Congress.

At the same time, private insurance companies began to list covered and noncovered services and procedures in their summary plan descriptions.

Further moves to define medical necessity have remained stagnant for some time. Private insurers continually use the term as a means to direct the review of any claim, which can be a prospective, concurrent, or retrospective review. These same companies have added another layer to medical necessity by publishing internal guidelines on what are or are not covered items and relegating them under the umbrella of a medical necessity review. These guidelines are most often based on each company's own research of evidence-based medicine, but, as a point of interest, they seldom include research conducted in other countries, which limits the scope of accepted practice. What one company deems investigational under its medically necessary care may have been a prescribed treatment regime in other countries for years.

Medicare and medical necessity

Medicare has published its latest version of medical necessity in the *Medicare Benefit Policy Manual* (Pub 100-02). It is defined not in terms of medically necessary care but in terms of who inpatients are and how physicians must judge who is to be admitted. Medicare defines inpatients as follows:

> An inpatient is a person who has been admitted to a hospital for bed occupancy for purposes of receiving inpatient hospital services. Generally, a patient is considered an inpatient if formally admitted as inpatient with the expectation that he or she will remain at least overnight and occupy a bed even though it later develops that the patient can be discharged or transferred to another hospital and not actually use a hospital bed overnight.

> The physician or other practitioner responsible for a patient's care at the hospital is also responsible for deciding whether the patient should be admitted as an inpatient. Physicians should use a 24-hour period as a benchmark—that is, they should order admission for patients who are expected to need hospital care for 24 hours or more and treat other patients on an outpatient basis. However, the decision to admit a patient is a complex medical judgment that can be made only after the physician has considered a number of factors, including the patient's medical history and current medical needs, the types of facilities available to inpatients and to outpatients, the hospital's bylaws and admissions policies, and the relative appropriateness of treatment in each setting. Factors to be considered when making the decision to admit include such things as:

- The severity of the signs and symptoms exhibited by the patient;

- The medical predictability of something adverse happening to the patient;

- The need for diagnostic studies that appropriately are outpatient services to assist in assessing whether the patient should be admitted (i.e., performing the studies does not ordinarily require the patient to remain at the hospital for 24 hours or more);

- The availability of diagnostic procedures at the time when and at the location where the patient presents.

According to Medicare:

> Admissions of particular patients are not covered or are noncovered solely on the basis of the length of time the patient actually spends in the hospital. The intermediary does not deny an admission that includes covered care, even if noncovered care was also rendered. Under PPS, Medicare assumes that it is paying for only the covered care rendered whenever covered services needed to treat and/or diagnose the illness were in fact provided. If a noncovered procedure is provided along with covered nonroutine care, a DRG change rather than an admission denial might occur. If noncovered procedures are elevating costs into the cost outlier category, outlier payment is denied in whole or in part.

(Medicare Benefit Policy Manual, *Pub 100-02, pp. 4-1–4-2, Aug. 2005*)

The outlined terms lead one to believe that the judgment of the physician is the determining factor to meet medical necessity for admission and to prevent a denial. In general practice, a physician's judgment is generally insufficient if it is not accompanied by documentation of a potential adverse outcome and the description of a patient's clinical status as acutely ill and receiving treatment at an acute level of care. How a physician or a case manager should document the patient's clinical status in the medical record will be covered in depth in later chapters.

ERISA and SPD

An additional source of information on how to define medical necessity can be found in the Employee Retirement Income Security Act (ERISA) regulations. ERISA required companies that provide insurance for purchase by their employees to generate a summary plan description (SPD) that contains information on how the plan works, how to file a claim, what services are covered and noncovered, and how determinations are made, to name a few of the standards. Within most SPDs, there is generally a section on medical necessity. The following is typical information contained in SPDs:

Medically necessary (medical necessity)

The determination of medical necessity is made by the applicable healthcare company. Care is considered medically necessary if it:

- Is accepted by the healthcare profession in the United States as appropriate and effective for the condition being treated

- Is based upon recognized standards of the healthcare medical specialty involved

- Represents the most appropriate level of care: the frequency, duration, and site of services, depending on the seriousness of the condition being treated (e.g., in the hospital or in the physician's office)

- Is not experimental or investigative

The need to define medical necessity grew into a new resource business. Around 1972, the need to define medical necessity for admission and continued stay created a need for a standardized set of guidelines, or criteria, on which the decisions could be made. Rather than having a specific hospital-based nurse review the admission and make an arbitrary decision, companies began to collect data and review accepted standards. InterQual criteria, among some other small or legacy criteria sets, began to be used. It was important for case managers to have some backing in the review process when making a determination that a specific patient did or did not meet admission criteria. Physicians were still involved in the process, but it was very important to have a neutral guide, or criteria, on which to base decisions.

Most insurance companies follow these definitions, but now add the use of criteria sets (e.g., InterQual or Milliman Care Guidelines) under the guise of establishing medical necessity derived from evidence-based medicine and research.

Perhaps in the future, if medicine in the United States becomes more uniform, a standardized definition will exist, and as such, those who deal with medical necessity denials and those who wish to prevent denials will have a working definition of medically necessary care regardless of where they come from. In the meantime, it is essential to use the definition of medical necessity as delineated by the authority that you rely on for reimbursement and work within that parameter. Chapter 3 will discuss detailed methodologies on how to apply medical necessity criteria to prevent and overturn denials.

Hospital-Based Case Management

Case management has been in existence in the hospital setting for more than 20 years. New England Medical Center in Massachusetts is among those credited with establishing the first case management model. The medical center was able to develop a clinical case management approach by using CareMaps, which had well-defined patient interventions from admission to discharge (Roggenkamp, White, and Bazzoli, 2005). From that original hospital model a variety of practices have been developed. A review of the literature reveals that no consistent definition of a case management model exists, but rather that many organizations have used a combination of organizational structures and models.

The initial impetus to create a hospital-based case management department was primarily driven by cost. Case management has been in existence since the early 1900s with social programs and progressing to insurance companies to assist in cost containment. The hospital case manager (CM) position had its roots in both areas, as well as being propagated due to institutional influences to achieve the same level of success as a facility's competitors. Hospital CMs now focus on many areas that include a "collaborative process that assesses, plans, implements, coordinates and evaluates the options and services required to meet an individual's health needs using communication and available resources to promote quality and cost-effective outcomes" (Powell and Ignatavicius, 2001, p. 3). Within the current practice, hospital CMs have progressed to specialized areas within their scope of practice to include disease- or population-specific practice, utilization review (UR), discharge planning, clinical documentation, and coding, among others.

In the United States today, emergency departments (ED) face unprecedented challenges. Increased volume, consumer expectations and publically reported scorecards, regulatory compliance, insurance coverage determinations, and fiscal responsibility are among the myriad obstacles that must be navigated for EDs to be considered successful. The new paradigm of customer expectations for high-quality care in a setting that allows for quick turnaround, while not missing vital information, can put a strain on the capabilities of any well-run ED. The question that EDs across the country are asking is how to manage the challenges and be fiscally successful. One solution that many are implementing is ED case management. Case management has been a successful part of the hospital setting. In the past decade there has been an increase in the number of facilities using case management in the ED. The 2009 *American Case Management Survey* reported that 83%–85% of facilities with bed capacity from 200 beds to more than 500 beds had ED case management. Of those reporting that they do provide case management in the ED, there was a lack of dedicated emergency room case management and only an average 52% cover on Saturdays and 46% on Sundays both had 91%–95% responsibility to assist in other areas of the hospital.

Why have EDs moved to use case management? The benefits are numerous. Some of the advantages are in the ability of the CM, using the UR process and criteria, working with physicians to determine appropriateness of admission to acute inpatient status or to suggest admission to outpatient observation service, and assessing patients for post-discharge needs prior to inpatient admission. All of these processes support meeting compliance to standards of practice such as The Joint Commission, and Centers for Medicare & Medicaid Services (CMS), and the Social Security Act's Condition of Participation that the discharge process begin at admission. Working to avoid medically unnecessary or inappropriate admissions is the first step in preventing denials. ED case management involves monitoring patients who are frequently readmitted, sometimes referred to as "frequent flyers." This critical intervention can be a valuable link to community resources. Identifying patterns and trends in the use of ED services can lead to quality improvement efforts that are also among the duties of the ED CM.

Discharge planning

Discharge planning is essential to the role of any successful hospital. Postacute care planning is needed to maintain a length of stay (LOS) that is consistent with severity and case mix. Financial stability comes from managing utilization and patient days. In the ED, this translates to ensuring that a CM obtains vital data that start the discharge process. Opportunities to communicate with family members or the healthcare proxy may be lost or delayed once the patient is admitted, thus delaying the discharge process. As Bristow and Herrick noted, "The process of case management focuses on the coordination of healthcare services to facilitate cost-effective, positive patient outcomes. Having patients and family members actively participate in the planning process enhances compliance with the discharge plan" (2002). The ED

CMs can assess for placement issues and durable medical equipment or home health needs, thus assisting the in-house CM in the discharge process. The ED CM can also assist in placing patients directly from the ED without the need for a costly inappropriate admission, which leads to the prevention of a denial. Proactive discharge planning drives throughput and assists with LOS. Early identification of patient needs and the expected LOS can influence the expectations of the patient, family, and medical team to meet the clinical goals for treatment. The information gathered can also influence the case management care plan.

Utilization review

UR is a cornerstone of ED case management. As gate-keepers, CMs have knowledge of admitting criteria and can assist the ED physician in making the determination for placement. As noted by Romania, "Case managers can assist admitting physicians with identifying patients that do not meet acute care admission criteria. Once this is determined, efforts are then made to seek out the appropriate level/place of care for the patient" (2006). Placement in skilled nursing homes, psychiatric facilities, drug and alcohol rehabilitation, and shelters are among the discharge locations that a CM can assist with, thereby preventing unnecessary admissions and increasing throughput by saving a bed for those meeting admission criteria. This also helps prevent an admission denial and lack of reimbursement.

Observation status and the RAC

The ability to review admissions leads to savings because it enables placement of the patient at the correct level of care. Using observation service for those patients who meet the criteria can save the hospital money by decreasing denials. As Gautney et al. noted, "Each year nationally, about 600,000 chest pain patients are admitted to the hospital for inpatient care and are later diagnosed without any significant disease" (Gautney, Stanton, Crowe, and Tracey, 2004). With a new focus through recovery audit contractor (RAC) reviews, the need to properly admit patients is more crucial to keep the reimbursement that was billed. One- and three-day and inappropriate admissions are on the RAC radar. The days of not using observation service because Medicare only reviews 50 charts per month is over. RACs can go three years in their review and will issue denials for improperly admitted patients. Thus, the chest pain patient who should have been a one-day observation stay but who instead had a full admission and workup will be reviewed and result in a potential denial. Other diagnoses and symptoms fit the category of inappropriate admissions, such as abdominal pain, headaches, the so-called "failure to thrive," and the infamous "unsafe to discharge." Bringing a patient in for a three-day qualifying stay to access the Medicare Extended Care Benefit without meeting admission criteria also places the facility at risk for a denial. A pattern of this practice may also be reviewed for quality of care and potential fraud allegations. This is where the CM can intervene for placement directly from the ED. The ED CM can gather the necessary information for discharge planning if the patient is admitted and place the patient into the correct admission status to ensure correct reimbursement.

Many hospital financial departments are leery of using observation services due to the minimal reimbursement that goes along with it. The risk-reward benefit of placing the patient into a full admission was on the reward side due to the lack of audits conducted by Medicare. However, RAC audits have changed the landscape of the reviews being conducted by Medicare. A report published on the RAC demonstration project in February 2008 states that 3.9% of the Medicare dollars paid did not comply with one or more Medicare coverage, coding, billing, or payment rules. That equates to $10.8 billion in Medicare fee-for-service (FFS) over- and underpayments. In 2006, Congress required that the U.S. Department of Health and Human Services make the RAC program permanent and nationwide no later than January 1, 2010.

Fiscal integrity

Improper payments can occur in the Medicare FFS program when payments are made for services that were not medically necessary or did not meet the Medicare medical necessity criteria for the setting where the service was rendered.

In 2007, $99.2 million in payments were retracted following the RAC audits from inpatient hospitals in New York. Heart failure and shock accounted for $7.8 million of the overpayments collected by the RAC audits.

How can case management assist with the RAC? Reviewing admissions for proper inpatient or observation status and placement is key to decreasing the risk of a medically unnecessary denial. The ED CM should be an expert in admitting criteria, whether InterQual, Milliman, or national coverage determinations, as well as being able to articulate this to the admitting physician. A bond must be created within the ED to ensure that the ED CM is apprised and involved in the admission process.

"Frequent flyers" consume a lot of ED resources. A patient usually is tagged as a frequent flyer if he or she has three or more visits per month. Assumptions are sometimes made about the frequent-flyer patient because of the nature of the relationship that is created by the frequent visits. However, many of these patients have several comorbidities, poor living conditions, addictions, and afflictions that undermine their health, often coupled with an inability to seek and get care outside of the ED. Effective ED CMs will be able to intervene by exploring community-based resources, making clinic appointments, helping to secure financial assistance, and providing education. Although further investigation is needed to positively state that ED case management is a benefit, case management interventions have proven to decrease readmissions. Thus, it can be stated that interventions in the ED as listed earlier can lead to similar results.

Hospital case management will continue to develop, and facilities must stay abreast of regulatory changes that can impact the financial health of the institution. Economic forces are currently making all healthcare facilities in the United States reevaluate their processes to cut or eliminate cost. Emphasis should be on reduction of potential revenue loss. Preventing denials through the use of hospital CMs is one method facilities can use to do this.

The Birth of Evidence-Based Criteria

Prior to the development of criteria that supported decision-making in regard to who to admit and when to discharge, the discretion fell solely on the treating physician. Because there was no oversight, admissions, discharges, and LOS varied across geographical areas as well as between physicians.

With the establishment of Medicare came regulations such as "each provider organization was required to have an admissions committee to review medical necessity of admission, the length of stay, the discharge practice and the necessity of the services requested by the physician" (Mitus, 2008).

At the time Medicare began the regulations, providers turned to the *Professional Activity Study* (*PAS*) book, which was a compilation of data from medical record information that was computerized and received through a voluntary exchange. The information gathering began in 1953. The *PAS* had three components: basic data, patient care data, and optional concurrent review data used for UR. The optional data elements were number of days spent in care units, whether consulting physicians were used, and the total charges for the hospitalization (Mullener and Kobrinski, 1983). It was from these data that hospitals began to look at comparative LOS data. However, guidelines for best practice were lacking. The information provided was simply historical in nature and did not have benchmarks.

Other limitations of the *PAS* included the collection of the data and the analysis based on coding that was not uniform, creating discrepancies as high as 43% mostly based on the selection of the primary diagnosis (Luft, 1983).

At the time that *PAS* was being used, other companies were developing and selling criteria to assist in utilization decisions. In addition, an amendment in 1972 to the Social Security Act authorized the creation of professional standards review organizations (PSRO), which were set up to cut costs and to monitor medical necessity and improve the quality of the care being provided. Public Law 92-603 stated in section 249F that PSROs be set up "in order to promote the effective, efficient and economical delivery of heath care services of proper quality for which payment can be made, in whole or in part, under the Social Security Act ... " (*California Medicine, 39*).

In 1973, a nurse named Joanne Lamprey, along with attorney Charles Jacob and a physician, responded to a government request for proposal for assistance in developing a quality assurance program. Lamprey's work as a UR nurse allowed her to recognize the failures of the *PAS* and the need to create better criteria for UR. Jacob had been working with The Joint Commission when he met Lamprey, and shortly thereafter started what would become InterQual. They published their first set of criteria for *Severity of Illness and Intensity of Service* in 1978 (Mitus, 2008).

During this time frame, the HMO Act of 1973 was established with the hopes of decreasing cost, but in essence it raised cost to individuals.

The proliferation of managed care organizations (MCO) in general, and HMOs in particular, resulted from the 1965 enactment of Medicare for the elderly and Medicaid for the poor. Literally overnight, on July 1, 1966, millions of Americans lost financial responsibility for their healthcare decisions. Offering free care led to predictable results. Because Congress placed no restrictions on benefits and removed all sense of cost-consciousness, healthcare use and medical costs skyrocketed. Congressional testimony reveals that between 1965 and 1971, physician fees increased 7% and hospital charges jumped 13%, whereas the consumer price index rose only 5.3%. The nation's healthcare bill, which was only $39 billion in 1965, increased to $75 billion in 1971.

As patients have since discovered, the HMOs—staffed by physicians employed by and reporting to corporations—were not much of an improvement in the management of healthcare delivery. HMOs sell coverage of services, but because of the criteria established for appropriateness of coverage, they often deny coverage or access to the listed benefits. HMOs, like other prepaid managed care products, require enrollees to pay in advance for a long list of routine and major medical benefits, whether the healthcare services are needed, wanted, or ever used. The HMOs manage care and control and determine access to healthcare service through definitions of medical necessity, restrictive drug formularies, and HMO-approved clinical guidelines (Blaise, 2001).

PSROs have evolved into quality improvement organizations (QIO), and HMOs and PPOs have propagated to include Medicare Advantage plans, each with their own review process, guidelines, and evidence-based criteria to determine the medical necessity of a patient's care. As proof of the proliferation of evidence-based criteria guidelines, one of the largest and most successful QIOs, the Island Peer Review Organization *(www.ipro.org)* in New York, uses Milliman Care Guidelines *(www.careguidelines. com)* as a screening tool to provide guidance on when and who to admit, as well as where to discharge patients.

The quandary for hospitals is that there is more than one set of criteria, each with their pros and cons. One of the biggest cons is the cost associated with leasing the guidelines. Few hospitals can afford to have more than one set of criteria and therefore run the risk of incorrectly interpreting medical necessity based on the insurance provider's choice. Evidence-based research is a valuable tool in providing care that is proven to work, but when that same evidence is used to deny reimbursement, those in a position to stop and or appeal a denial can find themselves grasping for guidance on how to proceed. Throughout the next chapters, you will learn methods for decreasing the potential for a denial, how to use the evidence-based guidelines in a beneficial manner, and when to appeal with the use of those guidelines.

Summary

Medical necessity is the foundation of denial prevention. Understanding the history and significance of the terms that outline the criteria used by insurance companies, regulatory bodies, and government entities is crucial in establishing a denial prevention program and having the ability to overturn denials on appeal.

REFERENCES

1. AMA, *Policy H-320.953: Definition of "Screening" and "Medical Necessity."*

2. *Beal v Doe* 432 U.S. 438 (1977).

3. Bergthold, L. A. "Medical necessity; Do we need it?" *Health Affairs* Vol 14, No 4 (1995): 180.

4. Blanchard, P. "Medical Necessity Determinations: A Continuing Healthcare Policy Problem," *Journal of Health Law* Fall 2004: 601–602.

5. Brase, T. "Blame Congress for HMOs," *The Freeman: Ideas on Liberty* Feb 2001: 1.

6. Bristow, D., Herrick, C., "Emergency Department Case Management: The Dyad Team of Nurse Case Manager and Social Worker Improve Discharge Planning and Patient and Staff Satisfaction while Decreasing Inappropriate Admissions and Costs: A Literature Review" *Lippincott's Case Manager,* Lippincott Williams & Wilkins, Inc., Vol 7, No 3 (2002): 243-251.

7. *California Medicine, The Western Journal of Medicine,* 39.

8. Luft, H. "The Professional Activity Study of the Commission on Hospital and Professional Activities: A User's Perspective," *Health Services Research* Vol 18, No 2 (Summer 1983, Part II): 349–352.

9. Mitus, J. A. "The Birth of InterQual, Evidence-Based Decision Support Criteria that Helped Change Healthcare," *Professional Case Management* Vol 13, No 4 (2008): 228–233.

10. Mullener, R. and E. J. Kobrinksi. "The Professional Activity Study of the Commission on Professional Hospital Activities," *Health Services Research* Vol 18, No 2 (Summer 1983, Part II).

11. *Pinneke v Preisser* 623 F 2d 546, 550 (1980).

12. Powell, S. K. and D. Ignatavicius. *CMSA's Core Curriculum for Case Management*, Philadelphia: Lippincott Williams & Wilkins, 2001: 3.

13. Roggenkamp, S.D., White, K.R., Bazzoli, G.J. "Adoption of Hospital Case Management: Economic and Institutional Influences," *Social Science & Medicine* Vol 60 (2005): 2489–2500.

Utilization Review and Guidelines

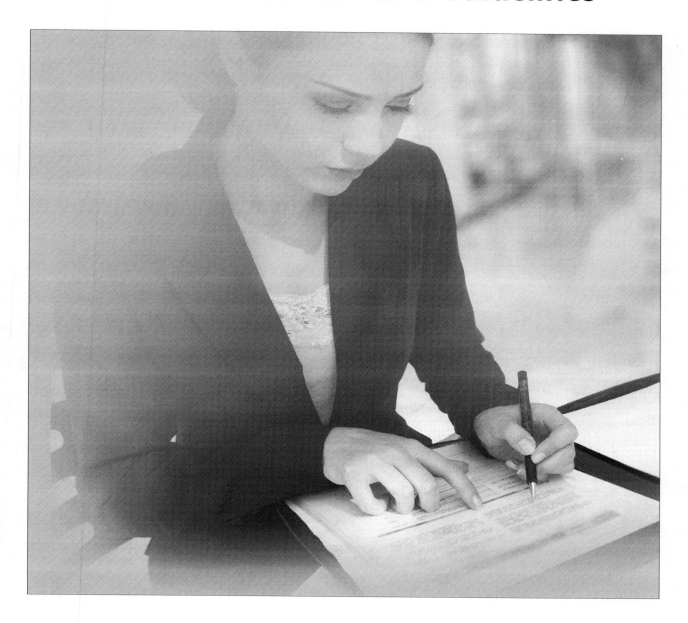

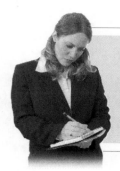

Utilization Review and Guidelines

Utilization Review Defined

Utilization review (UR) is the process by which medical necessity is established using a systematic approach based on a set of criteria, standards of care, guidelines, or other methodologies in which a patient's care is approved for reimbursement.

The basis for UR is to ensure that care delivered to patients is appropriate for time and setting and to control cost that will, in the end, provide sufficient monies to allow for care to be provided to all constituents.

UR can be conducted by various entities, including governmental agencies, contracted agencies, quality improvement organizations (QIO), private payers, and hospital committees. Most states also have a review process for Medicaid beneficiaries who can be reviewed by QIOs, contracted parties, and insurance departments of the state under public health or insurance laws.

Regulations that Support Hospital-Based UR

The federal government under the Social Security Act and the Centers for Medicare & Medicaid Services (CMS) *Conditions of Participation (CoP)* include the following provisions establishing hospital-based UR:

LEARNING OBJECTIVES

At the end of this chapter, the reader should be able to:

✔ Define utilization review (UR)

✔ State the regulation that supports need for hospital-based UR

✔ Discuss the differences between hospital UR and insurance-driven UR

✔ Name sources of evidence-based medicine

✔ Relate how criteria guidelines are derived

✔ Find evidence-based research articles to support UR

- Section 1861(k) of the Social Security Act provides the regulation for hospital-based UR

- CMS' *CoP* under title 42 of the *Code of Federal Regulations (CFR)*.

- Under the interpretive guidelines, exceptions to the UR committee are explained in 42 *CFR* 456.50 - 456.245

Section 1861(k) of the Social Security Act
Part E—Miscellaneous Provisions
Definitions of Services, Institutions, etc.[442]

Utilization Review

(k) A utilization review plan of a hospital or skilled nursing facility shall be considered sufficient if it is applicable to services furnished by the institution to individuals entitled to insurance benefits under this title and if it provides—

   (1) for the review, on a sample or other basis, of admissions to the institution, the duration of stays therein, and the professional services (including drugs and biologicals) furnished, (A) with respect to the medical necessity of the services, and (B) for the purpose of promoting the most efficient use of available health facilities and services;

   (2) for such review to be made by either (A) a staff committee of the institution composed of two or more physicians (of which at least two must be physicians described in subsection (r)(1) of this section), with or without participation of other professional personnel, or (B) a group outside the institution which is similarly composed and (i) which is established by the local medical society and some or all of the hospitals and skilled nursing facilities in the locality, or (ii) if (and for as long as) there has not been established such a group which serves such institution, which is established in such other manner as may be approved by the Secretary;

   (3) for such review, in each case of inpatient hospital services or extended care services furnished to such an individual during a continuous period of extended duration, as of such days of such period (which may differ for different classes of cases) as may be specified in regulations, with such review to be made as promptly as possible, after each day so specified, and in no event later than one week following such day; and

   (4) for prompt notification to the institution, the individual, and his attending physician of any finding (made after opportunity for consultation to such attending physician) by the physician members of such committee or group that any further stay in the institution is not medically necessary.

The review committee must be composed as provided in clause (B) of paragraph (2) rather than as provided in clause (A) of such paragraph in the case of any hospital or skilled nursing facility where, because of the small size of the institution, or (in the case of a skilled nursing facility) because of lack of an organized medical staff, or for such other reason or reasons as may be included in regulations, it is impracticable for the institution to have a properly functioning staff committee for the purposes of this subsection. If the Secretary determines that the utilization review procedures established pursuant to title XIX are superior in their effectiveness to the procedures required under this section, he may, to the extent that he deems it appropriate, require for purposes of this title that the procedures established pursuant to title XIX be utilized instead of the procedures required by this section. (Source: *www.socialsecurity.gov/OP_Home/ssact/title18/1861.htm#act-1861-k, accessed March 18, 2009.*)

CoPs by CMS
Title 42 - Public Health

Chapter IV - Centers for Medicare & Medicaid Services, Department of Health and Human Services
Subchapter G - Standards and Certification
Part 482 - Conditions of Participation for Hospitals
Subpart c - Basic Hospital Functions

482.30 - Condition of Participation: Utilization review.

The hospital must have in effect a utilization review (UR) plan that provides for review of services furnished by the institution and by members of the medical staff to patients entitled to benefits under the Medicare and Medicaid programs.

(a) Applicability. The provisions of this section apply except in either of the following circumstances:

(1) A Utilization and Quality Control Quality Improvement (QIO) has assumed binding review for the hospital.

(2) CMS has determined that the UR procedures established by the State under title XIX of the Act are superior to the procedures required in this section, and has required hospitals in that State to meet the UR plan requirements under Sec. 456.50 through 456.245 of this chapter.

(b) Standard: Composition of utilization review committee. A UR committee consisting of two or more practitioners must carry out the UR function. At least two of the members of the committee must be doctors of medicine or osteopathy. The other members may be any of the other types of practitioners specified in Sec. 482.12(c)(1).

(1) Except as specified in paragraphs (b)(2) and (3) of this section, the UR committee must be one of the following: (i) A staff committee of the institution; (ii) A group outside the institution (A) Established by the local medical society and some or all of the hospitals in the locality; or (B) Established in a manner approved by CMS.

(2) If, because of the small size of the institution, it is impracticable to have a properly functioning staff committee, the UR committee must be established as specified in paragraph (b)(1)(ii) of this section.

Interpretive Guidelines, Exceptions to the UR Committee
(42 CFR 456.50 through 456.245.)

- The regulation permits two exceptions to the requirement for a hospital UR plan: (1) where the hospital has an agreement with a QIO under contract with the Secretary to assume binding review for the hospital or; (2) where CMS has determined that UR procedures established by the State under Medicaid are superior to the UR requirements for the Medicare program and has required hospitals in that State to meet the UR requirements for the Medicaid program at 42 CFR 456.50 through 456.245.

- With regard to the second exception, CMS would have to determine that UR procedures established by a State under Medicaid are superior to the UR requirements for Medicare. Currently no UR plans established by a State under Medicaid have been approved as exceeding the requirements under Medicare and required for hospital compliance with the Medicare UR CoP within that State. In the event that CMS approves a State's Medicaid UR process for compliance with the Medicare UR CoP, CMS will advise the affected State Survey Agency.

Because of the regulations, the establishment of a UR committee and a process ensuring the ability to review cases to make medical necessity determinations provides the impetus for any facility to acquire the necessary personnel to meet the regulations. Other regulatory bodies such as The Joint Commission, although not mandating a UR committee, have in place a section on discharge planning and will review the entire process including the need for a patient to be hospitalized and when the patient should be discharged. Without understanding how to review an admission and subsequent stay, the case manager (CM) or UR personnel could have a difficult time in demonstrating a proper discharge plan. The UR process should include review of medical information to drive clinical milestones necessary to communicate with the attending physician. This includes when the milestones have been reached and at what level of care the patient should be at any given time.

For example, a patient with pneumonia may be admitted as an inpatient per the review guidelines provided there is involvement of two lobes, concomitant diseases in need of treatment, the patient's age, and other factors. Patients with an admitting diagnosis of pneumonia will be placed on IV antibiotics, oxygen, and perhaps IV fluids. Some of these patients will easily transition to oral antibiotics within three days and no longer require oxygen, but some will need prolonged treatment and perhaps a discharge to a lower level of care, such as home healthcare or some form of skilled nursing with a short-term rehabilitation plan (a dual plan). Most CMs have the experience and knowledge to understand this simple case, but when the patient's clinical complexity is higher and the plan that the CM established is not followed, where then does the case manager turn to provide the necessary information to the attending physician for him or her to make an informed decision regarding the discharge plan?

 Prevent Denials and Win Appeals

Most UR criteria sets include discharge screens for use in determining a patient's medical stability or readiness for discharge and some include references that provide a suggested next level of care based on the patient's clinical trajectory. These references can act as a good resource for the CM. In this way, the regulations that require UR in the hospital setting are joined with the care of the patient and the discharge plan. The regulations also indicate that if there is a discrepancy between the attending physician and the UR reviewer, the UR committee has the right to determine medical necessity, issue denials to patients, and advise them of their rights to appeal. The goal of the regulations and case management practice is to foster open communication between the UR physicians and the attending physicians. Frequently, CMs have had to rely on the rules, laws, and findings published by the different governing bodies to assert their accountability to establish and follow protocols that will lead to reversals of denied cases by the different payer sources.

Hospitals are also required to have in place a UR plan to show how they will manage situations in which there are conflicting conditions. For example, a patient may be medically ready for discharge, qualify for the Extended Care Benefit for post-hospital skilled rehabilitation, but there is no skilled nursing facility (SNF) bed available for the patient. Since this has a significant impact on delay in discharge, the UR committee/team must be involved in the process to continue to search for a bed for the patient.

CMS has a document that is used by many hospitals as a basic UR plan. The "Hospital Manual" is located at: *http://www.cms.hhs.gov/Manuals/PBM/list.asp? listpage=1.*

(*Note:* This is a zipped file. When the file is opened, select the section that includes the numbers 290.)

Some excerpts from the document will help readers identify why medical necessity for services is blended with clinical judgment and availability of medically necessary postacute services. Spacing of the document has been changed from the original to allow for ease in reading.

Availability and appropriateness of other facilities and services (290.3)

In determining whether further inpatient hospital stay is medically necessary, UR committees are required to take into account the availability and appropriateness of other facilities and services. The following guidelines should be used by UR committees in general hospitals:

- Determining required level of care

- Home healthcare as an alternative to institutionalization

- Location of alternative facilities

- Patients' financial status and personal preference

Determining required level of care

If the committee believes that the patient no longer requires hospital care but could receive proper treatment in a SNF, it should determine whether there is a SNF-level bed available to the patient in a participating SNF or swing bed hospital in the area. If there is, the committee should find that further stay in the hospital is not medically necessary.

If the committee determines that no SNF-level bed is available to the patient in a participating skilled nursing or swing bed facility, it should find that continued stay in the hospital is medically necessary.

The basis for the decision should be documented in the committee records. The committee will advise the attending physician that its decision is based on the lack of availability of a SNF-level bed and that it is his responsibility to attempt, on a continuing basis (with the assistance of the hospital's social worker, etc.), to place his patient in a participating SNF-level bed as soon as such a bed becomes available.

If the UR committee determines that the patient requires services other than inpatient hospital or extended care services, such as custodial, outpatient, or home healthcare, it should find, without regard to the availability of such kinds of care, that further inpatient hospital stay is not medically necessary.

Covered inpatient hospital or extended care services should not be considered as an alternative to noncovered or noninstitutional services.

Home healthcare as an alternative to institutionalization

A patient who needs hospital or extended care services continually requires a level of care and a scope of services that can only be provided in an institutional setting. Only those institutions that meet the conditions of participation for hospitals and SNFs are qualified to provide them.

A patient who needs home health services requires a minimal level of services which does not call for the patient to be institutionalized. For example, an individual may require only a single service, such as physical therapy. If the UR committee finds that an individual requires only home health services, it should not recommend continued inpatient stay, even if the required services are not available to the individual because there is no agency in the community that can provide the services, or there is an agency but the individual has no home to which he can be discharged.

Location of alternative facilities

A UR committee will consider which facilities are available in the community or local geographic area in deciding whether the patient can be cared for effectively elsewhere.

It is not possible to define community or local geographic area with any precision. However, as a general rule, a community or local geographic area should not be defined in such a way as to require a patient to be taken away from his family and transported over great distances.

Patients' financial status and personal preference

A UR committee should not take into account a patient's ability to pay for services or his coverage or lack of coverage under the health insurance program in deciding whether continued hospital stay is medically necessary.

A patient's preference for one SNF over another, such as a preference for a sectarian facility over a nonsectarian facility, should not be taken into account by the committee. If SNFs are available but the patient's preferred facility is filled, the committee should find that further inpatient stay is not medically necessary.

 Prevent Denials and Win Appeals

Differences between Hospital UR and Insurance-Driven (Payer-Based) UR

Hospital UR can seem similar to insurance-driven UR. They share many of the same reasons for review, primarily to ensure that the patient is receiving appropriate care and that there is a correct status assignment so the care will be appropriately reimbursed. Other areas of similarity are in ensuring appropriate LOS and correct adherence to the level of care.

The differences between hospital- and payer-based UR mainly stem from the perspective of resource allocation. The insurance company is trying to ensure that the benefits purchased by members are appropriately used, and to preserve and distribute funds to secure payment for all of its beneficiaries. On the other hand, the hospital's UR process is focused on the care of the individual patient who is present in the facility. The focus of the payer and the hospital UR process is also to properly move patients along the continuum of care from one level to the next. The hospital works to maximize reimbursement, especially in the face of a diagnosis-related group payer source. Using UR methods, CMs can more diligently examine the need for an admission and a continued stay, as well as the proper placement for the level of care required. UR can also assist in resource allocation and timely use of the resources, such as tests that need to be performed to ensure proper LOS. The UR committee in the hospital can function in a similar role as the insurance company by reviewing suspect, or marginally appropriate, cases and issuing denials to patients, particularly for Medicare and Medicaid beneficiaries.

With the institution of the Recovery Audit Contractor (RAC) program, the hospital-focused review takes on a more important role, which will be discussed further later in this book. In the case of a RAC review process, more focus is put on preventing a denial than on an LOS or continued stay review.

Sources of Evidence-Based Medicine

Evidence-based medicine (EBM) has exploded onto the scene in most hospitals in the form of clinical guidelines. The two most prevalently used criteria for UR, InterQual and Milliman Care Guidelines, rely on EBM to publish their criteria. The question is, where does it come from and how can it be used to prevent or overturn a denial?

According to the Centre for Evidence-Based Medicine, "Evidence-based medicine is the conscientious, explicit, and judicious use of current best evidence in making decisions about the care of individual patients" (Sackett et al., 1996). Physicians and physician extenders often rely on such research to advance their practice. New methods, treatments, and surgeries are proved useful, safe, and efficacious by studying the method, drug, or intervention, and thus become everyday practice.

In the United States, many insurance companies rely on EBM to create clinical guidelines that are used in making UR determinations and will often use only research that has been conducted in the United States, thus ignoring important research that has been initiated in other countries.

InterQual and Milliman provide a rich source of evidence-based articles in their bibliographies. Other sources include Medline, PubMed, and CINHAL, and online search engines such as Google and Yahoo! can provide a list of research articles that can be used in

---

the practice of UR. In later chapters, you will see evidence of this method being used to compile an appeal. Most of today's hospitals have access to electronic libraries, where a search can be conducted to extract research that supports your position.

How Criteria Guidelines Are Derived

InterQual and Milliman use a variety of methods to create their guidelines. InterQual states that criteria are developed by McKesson's clinical research staff, which includes physicians, RNs, and other healthcare professionals. Many of McKesson's clinical staff members hold advanced degrees and case management certification. The clinical content is reviewed and validated by a national panel of clinicians and medical experts, including those in the community and academic practice settings, as well as within the managed care industry throughout the United Sates. The clinical content is a synthesis of evidence-based standards of care, current practices, and consensus from licensed specialists and/or primary care physicians (InterQual Level of Care Criteria, 2008).

McKesson's acknowledgment that evidence-based standards of care are used provides an avenue to use newer research that can open a door to reverse a denial. Since McKesson publishes its guidelines annually, many of the articles used to create the guidelines are updated, but consideration of the articles' review and publication and the fact that not all research is used provides you the opportunity to inform reviewers of a new or more recently updated finding that can sway their opinion in your favor.

Milliman states the following about its guidelines:

> The full-time clinical staff that produces the Milliman Care Guidelines adheres to the industry's most rigorous evidence-based methodology. Over 100,000 articles were reviewed during the guideline development process, while a Milliman Care Guidelines epidemiologist examines databases that cover a significant portion of the United States population in order to validate that these published research results are achievable in real-life situations; 14,000 of these references are currently being cited in the seven-product Care Guidelines series (Milliman Care Guidelines, 2009).

As with InterQual, Milliman acknowledges the fact that research-based EBM is the primary driver behind its criteria. But again, it only reviews its guidelines annually, leaving room for new EBM to be introduced.

How to Find the Article You Need

Most research begins with a methodology that incorporates what is known and then a hypothesis is formed. To prove the hypothesis, the researcher postulates a question or series of questions that must be proved or disproved. Referencing a specific example, here are the recommended steps to take to ascertain the validity of a hypothesis:

1. State what you are trying to prove (e.g., admission for heart failure for administration of Milrinone).

2. Check the bibliography in the criteria set being applied (in this case, it is InterQual; there are 11 articles/guidelines referenced from 1999 to 2006 with only one article on Milrinone from 2004).

3. Search for articles on the subject (Milrinone and hospital admission) using those words as search terms.

4. Conduct an online search to find articles that can support the need to admit a patient for treatment (in this example, Medline produced three useful articles).

After the articles are researched, including the one in the guideline, a review of the information demonstrated that Milrinone used for patients with heart failure reduced LOS as well as readmissions. By admitting the patient and providing the proper care, the patient benefits from a reduction of hospital admissions and stabilization of the heart failure. When postulating the need for admission on an appeal as well as to the cardiologist in the emergency room, the CM can reference EBM to back up her or his claims.

This is just one example of how to search for material that can make the difference between an accurate admission and or a reversal on a denial. Further examples will be presented in later chapters. Being proficient in obtaining information by using online databases can lead to a better formalized approach in preventing and recuperating denials.

Summary

In conclusion, utilization guidelines, regulations, and laws govern facilities in their approach to handling reviews and how to establish committees that can assist with the process. The ability to research EBM will help when writing an appeal. Chapter 5 will discuss the steps involved in creating an effective appeal letter.

REFERENCES

1. Milliman Care Guidelines: *www.careguidelines.com/whycg/ebm.shtml*, accessed March 2, 2009.

2. InterQual Level of Care Criteria. McKesson Corporation, 2008.

3. Sackett, D. L., W. M. Rosenberg, J. A. Gray, R. B. Haynes, and W. S. Richardson. "Evidence-based Medicine: What It Is and What It Isn't," *BMJ* 312 (1996) 7023: 71–72. PMID 8555924, *www.bmj.com/cgi/content/full/312/7023/71.*

Denial Prevention

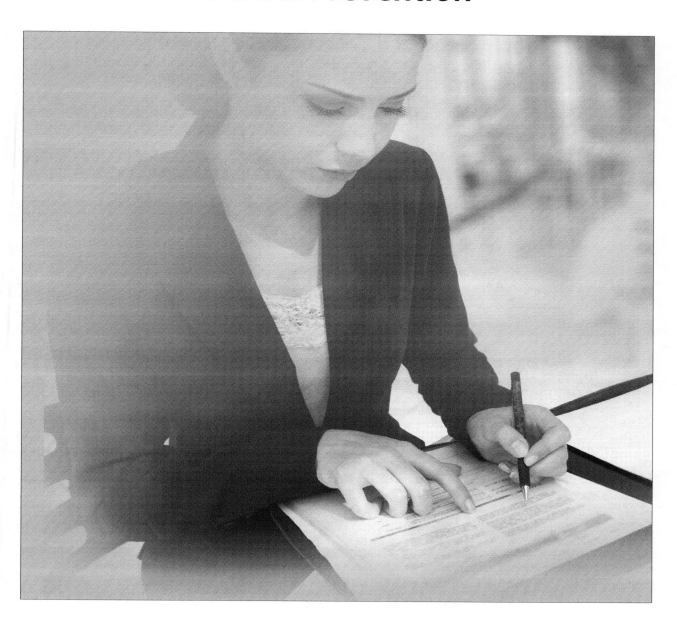

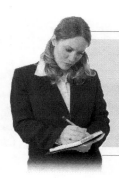

Denial Prevention

Denial Prevention Defined

Denial prevention is the ability to use a systematic approach to review admissions and continued stays to meet the definition of medical necessity. It includes helping the medical staff understand the importance of documenting the need for an acute care admission or continued stay and to provide orders that can be issued only by highly skilled staff members.

Most case management departments today understand the importance of preventing a medical necessity denial and can articulate the reasons behind its importance; however, what some departments do not understand is how to prevent denials and which resources should be allocated in the prevention. This chapter will discuss methods to achieve denial prevention and which resources can and should be allocated for the job.

Utilization review

In discussing denial prevention we should first note that activities surrounding initial utilization review (UR) lay the groundwork necessary to maximize the approval of admissions, thus preventing an admission denial. UR, as explained in the previous chapter, is the systematic process of review for medical necessity by whichever criteria are chosen to examine the need for an admission. In addition, the reviewer should also

At the end of this chapter, the reader should be able to:

✔ Describe denial prevention

✔ Execute denial prevention strategies

✔ State the role of the physician advisor in denial prevention

✔ Identify strategies to track denial prevention

be aware of the criteria used by the patient's primary and, sometimes, secondary payer, whether Medicare, Medicaid, or another payer source. The need to understand the payer source is most evident by the various states in which Medicaid does or does not acknowledge an admission to observation service. Agreements between the hospital and other payer sources can also affect the status to which the patient can be admitted. Most private payer sources will only pay for observation for a 23- to 24-hour

Prevent Denials and Win Appeals   © 2009 HCPro, Inc.   **29**

stay, depending on the agreement. CMs performing UR should have the opportunity to see a matrix of the payer sources to better understand how to complete

a UR. **Figure** 3.1 is an example of a payer matrix that can be used by CMs.

Payer	Criteria Used	Payment Structure
Medicare	Medicare regulations/InterQual	MS-DRG
Medicaid	Medicaid regualtions	DRG
BC/BS	InterQual	MS-DRG
Cigna	InterQual/Internal Policies	Mix-Per-diem and DRG
Aetna®	Milliman/Internal Policies	Per-Diem
Tricare	InterQual/Internal Policies	Mix-Per-diem and DRG

An understanding of the agreement is vital for the UR nurse to properly work with the patient's admitting physician in selecting the appropriate status to which to admit the patient to maximize reimbursement and prevent a denial.

Denial prevention begins when a patient enters the system; therefore, it is incumbent upon the case management department to examine where patients come from. For most facilities, this means the emergency department (ED), outpatient surgical areas, and direct admissions. For larger institutions and regional centers, transfers and clinics can add to the daily caseload. A review of volume of admissions per area can provide insight into the resources necessary for sufficient case management coverage to review admissions. Most initial reviews take 15–20 minutes depending on the knowledge and skill set of the reviewer, the criteria used, and whether a manual paper-based assessment or software assessment is

completed. Patients with complex situations, which include transfers, can take longer. When assessing for staffing resources to be allocated, consider the time of admission, throughput, volume, and the level of the reviewer's expertise.

Case mix

Another key area that should be analyzed is the case mix of patients. In organizations with a high percentage of managed care patients, there is a need to examine the patient's point of entry more carefully. This is required to obtain the maximum ability to ensure proper notification to the payer and ensure authorization for admissions. Most state insurance laws, along with federal regulations, allow time after an emergency admission—usually up to 24 business hours—to notify the insurance carrier of an admission; thus the review, if not completed at the point of entry, can be completed on the unit where the patient is placed. Best practice would avoid delay in notification and authorization by treating all patients equally for review purposes.

Medicare beneficiaries

With CMS starting the full RAC process, Medicare patients should have a review at the point of entry. Medicare provides an opportunity to use the advanced beneficiary notice (ABN) to inform and include the beneficiary in the decision for an admission if the necessary criteria are not met. According to CMS, the purpose of an ABN is to inform a beneficiary before he or she receives specified items or services that Medicare is unlikely to pay for on this particular occasion. CMS says, "The ABN allows the beneficiary to make an informed consumer decision whether or not to receive the items or services for which they may have to pay out of pocket or through other insurance" (Healthcare Financial Management Association, 2004).

By including the beneficiary in the discussions, the facility can potentially prevent a denial for an unnecessary admission. However, if the patient insists on the admission and the physician concurs, a preadmission denial may be issued, which provides the patient with the opportunity to have the quality improvement organization (QIO) review the admission and determine whether medical necessity for the admission meets local standards of care. The preadmission denial notice is rarely used. The QIO acts as a second opinion since it has a broader focus. Although the QIO cannot determine who is responsible for the reimbursement, it can answer the question asked by payers: Was this admission medically necessary? This process can occur only if there is a UR committee in place and an understanding of when to initiate the denial process.

Executing Denial Prevention

Denial prevention begins by establishing channels that lead to a systematic review of each patient's admission. A systematic review should include the history of the present illness, past medical history, current treatment, and the medical plan for continued treatment. In some situations social issues that can affect admission or discharge must be considered, particularly if the issues affect the patient's ability to receive necessary medical care. Prehospital treatment should be included, as it pertains to medical intervention by the patient's private physician or other medical personnel (e.g., a paramedic). Other resources are the documentation by the medical staff, contracting language, and regulations that assist in setting standards for reviews and execution of denial prevention.

Documentation

Documentation by the medical staff is one of the pillars that lead to reimbursement success. It can be argued that documentation is the singular issue in receiving a denial. At the end of this chapter is a case study that will demonstrate the need to educate physicians and their licensed extenders about how a denial can be prevented by documenting the true nature of the acute episode. Most physicians and their extenders are not trained to think in terms of denial prevention but rather in terms of how to document findings, symptoms, and signs, and what the plan of care will be. If it becomes necessary, the documentation should allow the reviewer to prove his or her case to an outside agency (e.g., the QIO responsible for determining the medial necessity and status of the admission).

Clinical documentation specialists

Many hospitals have turned to clinical documentation specialists (CDS) to assist in the improvement process to maximize reimbursement by increasing the case-mix index (CMI). CMI is a financial indicator of the complexity of the patient based on the documentation that leads to the final DRG coding. Each DRG carrier has a relative weight, which is established by Medicare on past years' discharges, which is then used in the calculation of the CMI. Although the CMI can add revenue, it does not necessarily translate into prevention of a denial. The CDS must work in collaboration with case management to meet the needs of coding and avoid denials. In executing a plan to prevent denials, CDSs and CMs should work in conjunction to educate the medical staff about the importance of describing the acute episode in such a manner that will unequivocally demonstrate that the patient cannot be treated at a lower level of care. Many CDS programs focus on disease states that can potentially be coded into a higher Medicare severity DRG (MS-DRG), thus providing a higher reimbursement rate. However, that can also falsely elevate the expected LOS and create missed opportunities to admit patients that commonly present for evaluation.

Contracting language

Hospitals enter into contracts with various payers, and the contracting language should be part of the prevention program. In the author's experience, managed care contracts sometimes include lower payment rates at a skilled level of care, sometimes called an alternate level of care or a lower neonatal ICU level. Hospitals would be well served to bring case management into the review of the proposed agreement prior to signing the contract. Case management should be involved in the contracting to ensure that medical necessity review language is included in the agreement, to the extent that the agreement follows state and federal regulations, and that information is shared on the methodology of the reviews along with timing, appeals, and rate structure. The author has reviewed contracts that contain a rate for a skilled nursing facility for high-risk pregnancies. Why should an acute care facility receive a reduced payment rate for a service that cannot be provided at a lower level of care? Many would argue that it is better to receive some payment than none at all, but if there is no place other than the acute care hospital to provide care, then the payer should pay for the services provided. If there is such a clause in a contract, the hospital should be in constant and detailed discussions with the insurance company's CM to help find a facility willing to take on that patient and provide the necessary care. These types of situations do not need to go to this extreme; this scenario is meant as an example only. However, the negotiation of the contract should be in the best interest of the patient, and pointing this out to the insurance company can only be done in the proper execution of a denial prevention program.

Regulations

Regulations such as the Employee Retirement Income Security Act (ERISA) and state insurance review laws, along with prompt payment laws, should also be included when rolling out the prevention program. Include language in the agreements that contain ERISA provisions (See Appendix B for the location of the full regulations). Consent forms should be tailored to provide an avenue for appeal without the need to obtain a separate consent to appeal. Consent forms should also provide an avenue to include third parties in the transmission of necessary information to obtain authorizations for care.

A well-executed plan will fit within the UR plan that is necessary under the *Conditions of Participation*, The Joint Commission standards, and many state laws. Having a clinical determination policy to reference is also part of the plan, but to maximize the potential of the program and achieve success, education of the case management staff, medical staff, executives, admissions, registration, health information management, nursing, and any other department that has a hand in the business side of patient care is necessary. Denial prevention does not exist in case management alone and must be shared by the parties listed here. To achieve buy-in for the necessary resources, a plan should demonstrate a return on investment. On the accompanying CD-ROM, there is a sample full-time equivalent justification that provides a blueprint to achieving success in allocating resources.

The Roles of the Physician Advisor

What is a physician advisor (PA) and why should you have one? A PA is a physician whose role is to work with and advise the CMs in UR in determining medical necessity. PAs should be an integral part of the case management department for many reasons: They can bridge the gap to the medical staff, provide support for review, act as a co-chair for the UR committee, and be a liaison in situations in which the advice of a clinical expert is needed to provide further information for a patient or family to give informed consent.

Many job descriptions and myriad roles exist for the PA. The PA should understand medical necessity and controlling LOS as a means to providing care to those in need and to assist in preventing the loss of revenue by unmonitored medical staff. As previously stated,

the days of the physician being in total control of the admission and discharge process has long passed. The PA can serve as the bridge to reluctant practitioners who still insist that they are in control and explain to the physician in his language the need to ensure the proper admission and discharge of his patients, which directly affects reimbursement.

PAs can help make a medical necessity determination after the initial review is complete if there is a question about the need for an admission or the level of care assignment. PAs' work should be tracked, including interventions that lead to changes in status assignment, approval of level of care, and assistance with discharges and overturning denials.

In preventing denials, the role of the PA should be to educate his or her peers on how to properly document a patient's level of illness and the treatment modality that demonstrates the acuteness of the illness to avoid denials. Physicians are more apt to listen to a peer than a CM until a good relationship is established; the PA can assist in this relationship development by being supportive of the case management role.

The availability and breadth of the PA role is usually dictated by the size of the facility, but it should be based on the necessary interventions. Even small facilities may find that, when initiating a prevention program, they require a full-time advisor to be a champion and assist in the fundamental culture change necessary to achieve success.

Choosing the right PA can be a difficult and lengthy process if there has never been one or if there have been weak advisors in the past. Ideally, the advisor should be a physician that has the respect of his or her peers, understands the business side of healthcare, and can articulate the importance of properly admitting and discharging patients to the best level of care and in the best interest of the patient. When interviewing a candidate, the case management/UR department should be involved, being careful not to base decisions on criteria knowledge alone. Anyone can be taught criteria who has the requisite foundation and is willing to learn.

Tracking Denials for Prevention

How do you measure success? The typical way is to establish a goal, set in place an action plan, and track the data to determine progress. Denials, like most issues in healthcare, should be tracked and trended over time to determine the level of success that is achieved. Many of the larger facilities and healthcare systems have software systems to assist in the task of tracking and trending. The most successful organizations involve quality management in the production of the data to demonstrate with a high level of confidence that the information is accurate so that it can be shared and defended as needed. For smaller facilities that do not have the IT budget to purchase software systems, there are examples on the CD included with this book that provide spreadsheets to track the data.

The big questions are: What should be tracked, how often, and by whom? The answers depend on the business model at your facility, but it is strongly advised that whoever is involved in the reviews should be able to receive reports on the denial percentage and what caused the denials. The following is a list of the most common elements to include in the tracking and trending:

- Patient demographics

- Insurance information

- Date and finding of initial and subsequent reviews with results (i.e., approved, not approved)

- Days approved

- Level of care approved

- Reviewer

- Attending physician

- MS-DRG

- Unit patient was on

- Service line

- PA involvement (second-level review, outcome)

- Date of denial

- Date denial received

- Appeal due date

- Date appeal sent

- Date appeal determination due

- Results of appeal and level of appeal (e.g., reversed, upheld, agreed, first or second level, external)

- Net revenue due

- Proposed amount

- Final payment

- Net gain or loss

Other items may be added for specific circumstances as needed. It is important to collect the data and, at a minimum, conduct a monthly review of the data to examine any trends. Control charts, which show a trend of information that includes control limits based on standard deviations, are ideal for determining whether variations are normal or special, or the level of order changes and can be produced in a manner that will demonstrate a high level of confidence in the statistical analysis and leave little or no room for argument.

Denial prevention is a cannon in the arsenal of methods that facilities can use to minimize underpayments and maximize reimbursement. Through the expertise of their staff, CMs are in the best position to lead the way in increasing profitability that can prove the worth of the case management department. By showing that case management can affect the bottom line while still providing the necessary clinical services to patients, CMs can strengthen its reputation as a respected department of any hospital regardless of size, payer mix, or patient population. Consider the case study on the following pages.

CASE STUDY

A 78-year-old white male presents to the ED Friday evening accompanied by his son who states that his dad has had an increase in the number of falls and an increase of confusion. His son says that his family can no longer care for him and want him admitted for placement in a nursing home. The physical exam reveals a well-nourished patient who has difficulty relaying the history of his illness; vital signs are within normal limits, and his baseline labs are slightly out of normal range but are not within the range that would indicate the necessity for admission based on the criteria set. The son provides information about the patient's history, including diabetes, hypertension, past history of a myocardial infarction, and recent escalation of confusion with an inability for self-care. The patient is living with his son, daughter-in-law, and their two young children. The patient's bedroom is on the second floor with a bathroom located on the same floor. He uses an assistive device to ambulate and until four weeks ago had not had any falls. In the past five days, there have been three falls, with one urgent care visit for bruising after a fall, with no fractures. A CT scan reveals degenerative changes but no acute process.

The physician orders a full inpatient admission for further evaluation and places the patient on telemetry to rule out any cardiac origin for the falls. He also orders an MRI/MRA, as well as an IV at 75cc/hr and routine labs in the morning. The patient has neurological checks every four hours and a check of routine vitals with I&O per shift. He is placed on a low-sodium diet, physical therapy (PT), and neurological consult with case management for discharge planning for placement.

After reviewing the information, the case manager (CM) makes the determination that the patient does not meet admission criteria; however, the physician disagrees, citing the son's wishes and agreeing with PT that the patient is unsafe to discharge.

The patient has fee-for-service Medicare Part A. In this extremely common scenario, the CM knows there is a high probability that Medicare will not pay for the stay, nor will the patient qualify for the needed three-day stay to be transferred to a nursing home.

The question that arises in this case is how to best approach the physician to provide documentation that will support an inpatient admission.

A review of the data shows that the patient has comorbidities that require self-medication to control the diabetes and the hypertension. The CM should approach the physician to document what would happen to the patient if discharged home, with emphasis on the probability of an adverse outcome. The CM knows that Medicare uses the predictability of an adverse outcome as one of the factors in determining

Prevent Denials and Win Appeals

the need for an admission, and therefore, he should coach the physician to state that, due to inability to provide self-medication, the patient's diabetes and hypertension will likely become out of control with the possibility of diabetic coma, diabetic keto acidosis, and a hypertensive crisis. In addition, the physician should document that the patient is in danger of further harm from the increased frequency of falls leading to fractures and potential death from traumatic injury, and that the cause of the recent increase in falls may be related to a cardiac condition which needs diagnosis and a treatment plan.

By documenting the preceding information, the physician establishes the patient's need to be cared for at an acute level of care for treatment and stabilization of the dementia and the initiation of PT, and to examine any other causes for the increased falls.

Such documentation will provide an avenue to argue the case for an acute level of care so that a safe discharge can be obtained.

In addition, the CM should discuss with the patient's son the possibility that Medicare will not pay for the admission. After reviewing the patient's situation with the ED physician or the physician advisor, an ABN can be provided to assist in the decision process. If the son and the beneficiary insist on the admission and the admitting physician agrees to admit, a preadmission HINN (hospital-issued notice of noncoverage) should be issued. If the son appeals, there will be documentation to support the admission, so the hospital places itself in the best situation for a win-win scenario. The CM should also begin the discharge process to seek out community-based resources that provide care in the home to potentially avoid a nursing home admission following the patient's stabilization and diagnosis. The plan should also include seeking short-term respite care, which is sorely needed by the patient's son.

Summary

Prevention begins by establishing a method of systematic review by CMs at the point of entry. The review encompasses the patient, the family, and the medical team's treatment and thoughts, as well as the documentation. Bringing the patient and the family into the equation can also prevent unnecessary admissions.

REFERENCES

1. Healthcare Financial Management Association. *Medical Necessity Denials: Prevention Pays Off.* Gale Group, 2004: 3.

Financial Impact

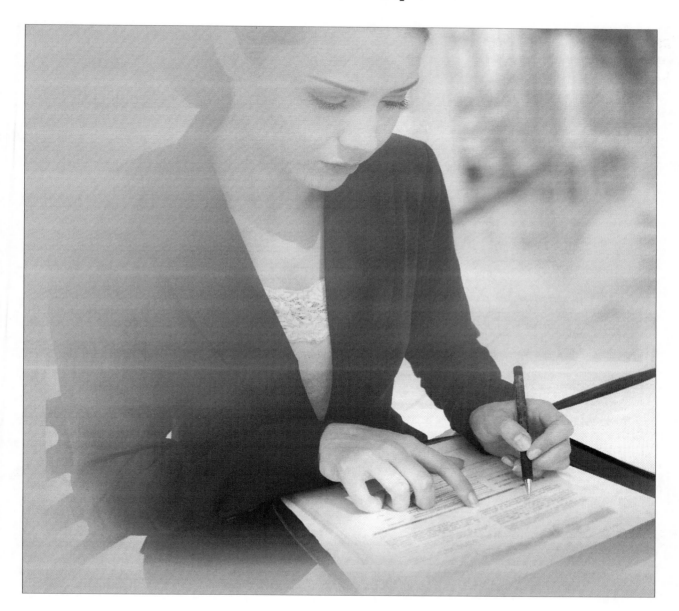

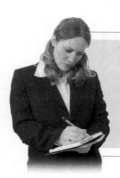

Financial Impact

The Revenue Cycle

For any institution, the revenue cycle is the lifeblood for maintaining profitability and ensuring that patients receive the services they seek in a cost-friendly manner. Imagine that when you were treated at Hospital A, your bill was double that of Hospital B. You would subsequently shop around for the less costly care with similar quality outcomes. Hospitals can charge only what is reasonable or they will not be able to stay profitable. Contracts dictate the charges that can be applied toward a patient's care along with federal and state reimbursement schemes. Many contracts state that the patient can be billed only for a small percentage of the care that is within the agreement between the hospital and the insurance company. Many of the contracted rates that are negotiated with payers include clauses to minimize the out-of-pocket costs for beneficiaries. This in return can help a plan becoming a preferred provider with access to the many lives covered by the health plan. The federal and state plans also have limits on billing patients.

The hospital has the responsibility to ascertain the proper billing information and to perfect the bill prior to being reimbursed, which includes ensuring that patients are treated according to medical necessity. All hospitals have some form of revenue cycle

LEARNING OBJECTIVES

At the end of this chapter, the reader should be able to:

✔ Discuss where case management and denial prevention fit within the revenue cycle

✔ Identify members of case management involved in the revenue cycle

✔ Identify how to partner with the finance department

✔ Calculate the savings and offset the losses of denials

management team, although they may vary in terms of process and participants. Best practice includes the following departments:

- Finance

- Patient access

- Collections

- Health information management, including coding

- Case management

- Executives

- Contracting

- Clinical representation

Having an individual from each of these areas will allow for pertinent discussion about issues affecting the flow of the revenue cycle. This can lead to process improvement without the need to convene individual meetings to discuss each issue. It is also recommended to include a medical or clinical leader such as the chief medical officer or the chief nurse executive. Any issue that delays the collecting, sharing, and verification of necessary information to be able to bill and receive proper payment for rendered services will affect the revenue cycle.

Where Does Case Management Fit in the Revenue Cycle?

The role for case management can be defined in terms of its area of expertise, which includes utilization review (UR), discharge planning, regulatory compliance related to reimbursement, and the use of those regulations to safeguard against unnecessary admission of patients. Through the advance beneficiary notice, Hospital-Issued Notice of Noncoverage, and the Important Message from Medicare process, case managers (CM) provide a critical oversight to appropriateness of care. Case management also has a role in the appeal of denials and the tracking and trending of denials that lead to process improvement.

Revenue cycle meetings discuss areas in which the hospital cannot collect or bill appropriately for services rendered.

Traditional revenue cycle management includes the expenditure of efforts and resources on the back end prior to the bill being dropped. Because CMs can prevent denials and are positioned to report on status issues, they can positively affect the ability to improve processes that lead to greater revenue capture in a timely manner. Laforge and Tureaud stated the following in *Heatlhcare Financial Management*, which describes the need to use a proactive approach within the revenue cycle:

> *The revenue cycle correlates strongly with the patient-flow process, which runs from scheduling and registration through treatment, discharge, and collection. In the past, hospitals tended to focus their efforts at the end of this process, on billing and collection. Yet most revenue-cycle problems originate early on, at the time when the hospital is collecting and verifying patient information needed to ensure submission of a clean claim and receipt of full payment. Rather than address problems retrospectively, hospitals should focus their efforts on front-end processes that help ensure the problems do not arise in the first place (Laforge, Tureaud, 2003).*

How Denials Affect the Revenue Cycle

Denials affect the revenue cycle by delaying the healthcare facility's ability to receive reimbursement in a timely manner, which increases the accounts receivable (AR) days and thus leads to monthly budgetary issues. If you consider reimbursement in terms of your paycheck, imagine that you will not be paid on time because an issue arose with the payroll department that takes up to six months to correct. A denial can take that long to get overturned if each level of appeal proceeds through the maximum time allowed under the law. RAC processes can take even longer if an appeal ends up in the administrative law judge's jurisdiction.

Not having your paycheck can render you unable to pay your bills and consequently damage your credit. The same holds true for a hospital. Some experts will assert that hospitals plan for that possibility, but what if there are more denials than budgeted or there is an economic downturn affecting the cash that was set aside for that situation or a disaster damages a system within the hospital and the cash on hand must

be used for capital expenditures? The same applies to denials if they go unchecked, and that is why attention to preventing them is on the radar of any competent chief financial officer (CFO).

A 5% denial rate at a moderate-size facility with 30,000 discharges per year can have an effect of more than $8 million on an average payment of $5,500. Having that much money in AR will negatively affect the hospital's ability to pay its creditors and stay in the black. Each 1% reduction in the denial rate for such an institution will lead to a capture of $1.6 million.

A well-run revenue cycle should resemble the example shown in **Figure 4.1**. Efforts to prevent denials will lead to greater operating revenue. Case management departments through UR, decreasing length of stay (LOS), and issuing denial letters to those who should

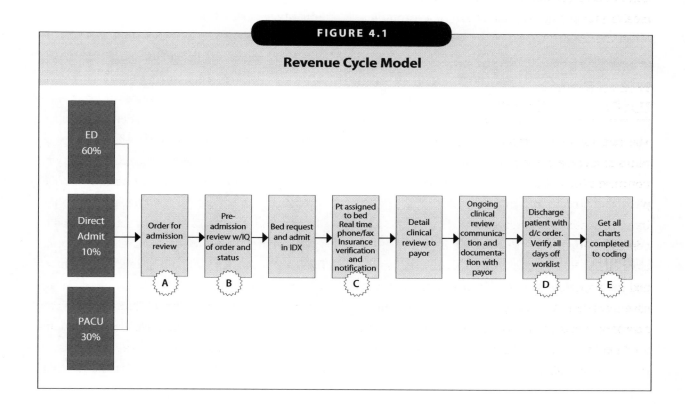

FIGURE 4.1

Revenue Cycle Model

not be admitted or stay in the hospital beyond the need for medically necessary continued stay, will have a positive influence on the revenue cycle.

Partnering with the Finance Department

Establishing ties to the finance department should be an endeavor that is pursued until accomplished. Case management has myriad ties to the financial status of any organization as outlined throughout this book. Being able to share information and provide data that affect the hospital's bottom line will open doors to resources. The CFO has the ability to approve or deny any program or resources with associated costs. Providing proof of case management's ability to prevent denials by properly assigning admission status, preventing inappropriate admissions, and discharging patients without delay days, will win your department allies and allow you to earn a prominent seat at the table for decision-making within your institution.

The data that are presented to any chief should be delivered in a manner that will prevent questioning of the data's validity. Control charts provide a means of delivering top-notch information that will unequivocally prove success or demonstrate stability or instability. Because of the construction of control charts, any trend can be acted upon with confidence that it is real and not illusory.

How to win friends in finance and garner support

Every day, CMs juggle duties to provide a method to allow patients to move through the continuum of care in the best manner possible. To achieve success, the staff builds on relationships with numerous stakeholders. The leaders in each institution have the dual role of protecting patients while maintaining a sound financial picture. The revenue cycle is just as important as the patient in care because of the ability to drive the cash flow of the hospital. The case management department is in the position to deliver real-time prevention of revenue loss. To build the relationships necessary to acquire the resources to meet the demand of an ever-changing financial picture, there must be collaboration with those who control the purse strings. Attending meetings and presenting data that have meaning to the financial team can lead to additional resources. To be persuasive, case management leaders must articulate the return on investment in financial terms, understand the pressures of the business office, and display the ability to be flexible when dealing with budgets and cost control. Using the qualities that are inherent in case management leaders, you should be able to influence without authority and use a transformation change approach to garner support for activities that will lead to increased revenue and resources.

Building working relationships with staff members in the business office, health information management department, with the finance officer, and revenue cycle team is just as important as building relationships with the medical staff and external resources when a CM advocates for a patient. To build those relationships, CMs must use their skills of negotiation, collaboration and leadership to meet the demands of the daily grind. Think about the negotiating that takes place among physicians and families to create an effective discharge plan and translate that skill set into doing the same with the revenue cycle team. It is that simple.

Reporting to Finance

Reporting to finance should include data that demonstrate the success of the case management department. The data that should be reported monthly include the overall denial rate for each denial category, length of stay, and avoidable days. The report should also include cost savings associated with the prevention of inappropriate admissions and prevention of delay days. Throughput, a term used to describe the ability to move a patient through the facility from admission to discharge, is essential to the success of any facility, as each patient who is seen is a potential admission. In most emergency departments, for every three patients seen, one is admitted. Some facilities have higher admission percentages. Without preventing inappropriate admissions, bottlenecks occur and denials start to pile up. Using proper UR procedures can help physicians admit proper patients to the proper areas, thus increasing throughput.

Severity of illness should also be reported. For example: InterQual publishes Severity of Illness/Intensity of Service criteria for acute care, making practical review of the appropriateness of hospitalization possible. If the case management department is safeguarding admissions, the severity should be as steady as possible. Most facilities have a mechanism for reporting severity of illness. If the severity has wide variability, an examination of UR and coding should occur.

Previously QIO organizations collected and distributed data through the Program for Evaluation Payment Patterns Electronic Report (PEPPER). These reports analyzed many of the common admissions that caused bottlenecks. The report of one-day stays, three-day stays, and most prevalent diagnosis-related groups (DRG) provided an avenue to analyze the effectiveness of the admission UR. The template of the PEPPER reports may be used by hospitals to recreate those data. The finance department will provide the data for you if you present the report you need, including the parameters to set up your own PEPPER reports. Collaboration with finance in this area will increase your value and allow you to stay on top of any issues that may start to get out of control or provide the information that will lead to improvement. To recreate a PEPPER report that will have an impact on preventing denials, you should track all one-day stays, three-day stays, and commonly denied DRGs. Using previous PEPPER reports analysis should take place to understand the areas of risk. After careful analysis, your new report should have only the data that are necessary to ensure compliance and to assist in maintaining vigilance on potential denial areas. In addition, the most commonly denied DRGs from RAC audits should also be tracked. Creating a dashboard that can be shared by the stakeholders can also lead to collaboration and cooperation to prevent denials.

Calculating Cost

There are many examples of the disparity of cost of care from one region to the next in the United Sates and even between hospitals in the same geographic area. The northeastern United States is known for the highest healthcare costs, whereas the Midwest is known for the lowest. This is due not only to taxes, but also to the population size and the overutilization of resources. Admitting a patient to the incorrect status can lead to denials and decreased revenue. At one facility at which the author worked, there was an average status error rate of about 3%. Per the director of coding from communication with other directors, the best hospitals were performing around the 1% rate. Low case-mix index also has a negative effect on revenue.

Many hospitals have turned to clinical documentation specialists (CDS), who have a high cost for small gains related to increasing revenue, but who assist in educating physicians on how to document properly. Although CDS staff members have success stories, the author believes that more evidence is needed to show the value and effectiveness of these programs. The change of DRGs to the Medicare severity DRG (MS-DRG) structure has led many hospitals to try to improve physician documentation to capture the highest category within the MS-DRG structure. This may artificially increase LOS and thus the cost of care. The decision of how to best admit and assign a patient to an admission status should be based on the medical necessity of the care rather than how well a physician can document congestive heart failure, for example. Most review criteria rely on the severity of the symptoms that can be demonstrated by the medical record, but the ability of the physician to document severity should be predicated on the patient's presentation and not on queries that inflate the MS-DRG category.

If the predicted LOS is inflated by better documentation coupled with a false sense of security of payment for the LOS, a decrease of payments due to length-of-stay denials or carve-outs on MS-DRG-based payers may result. Severity adjustment of LOS should be shared by the case management leadership along with the CMs and the medical staff so they can better understand trends. Trends should be correlated with any denials that affect payment at the back end of the stay. The cost of care at the end of the stay—that is, in the last few days of an admission—is generally lower than the start of the stay. However, for those who still have per diem payers, this is significant if the cost of care for each day during the admission exceeds the payment rate. Knowing the cost of care can also influence when to negotiate with external sources to prevent lengthy admissions. Effective and appropriate and patient-centered discharge planning will take advantage of networking with payers to negotiate the postdischarge cost of care rather than incur the cost in the hospital. Again the ability to move patients through the system in a timely manner will decrease the potential for a denial.

To calculate the cost of an admission, add the cost of care for each day of the stay and compare it to the payment of the MS-DRG or per diem rate to understand the revenue that is generated for each admission. The first three days of most admissions are generally the most costly due to the increased use of resources to examine, test, and treat the acute illness. The day of discharge is the least costly because of the decrease in utilization of resources.

Summary

Relationship building with the financial team will lead to added resources and place case management in a position of value. Data analysis and sharing will enhance the ability to provide information to drive process improvements. Become a partner in the revenue cycle even if you believe that most of the information presented does not relate to you. It does. Your ability to move cash and get paid for services rendered improves margins and increases viability for the facility.

REFERENCES

1. Laforge, R.W. (CPA) and J.S. Tureaud. "Revenue-Cycle Redesign: Honing the Details," *Healthcare Financial Management,* January 2003.

The Appeals Process

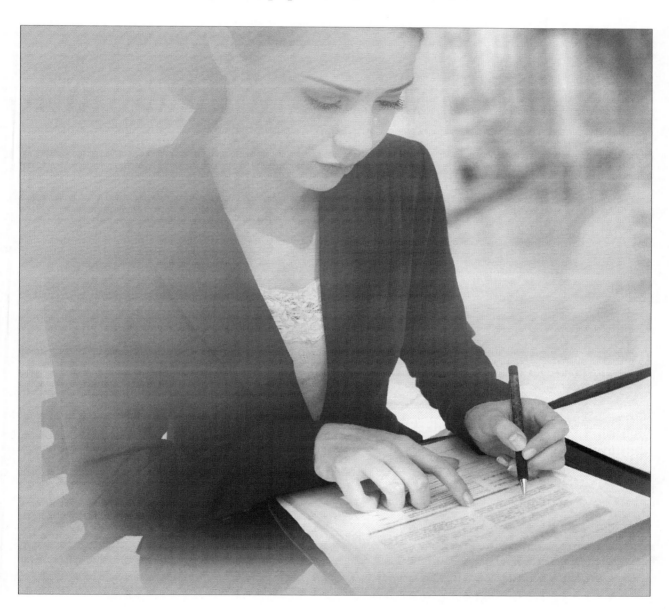

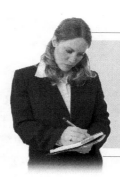

The Appeals Process

CHAPTER 5

Establishing a Baseline for Success Measurement

The appeals process can be an arduous task or it can be a flowing, evolving methodology that leads to success. Measurement of success for denial rates varies depending on the authority quoted. Within the discipline of case management, success can be measured by a rate of the percentage of denials against admission, patient days, discharges, and even against each payer source. In the author's experience, the level of success is measured by the dollars that were paid correctly against that which is expected.

As you measure the amount of your success or failure, you need to establish a baseline to measure the effectiveness of your denial prevention program. A typical denial rate is 2% or less minus Medicare and even Medicaid reviews. The true denial rate should be zero, but is that achievable? It should be, because denial prevention programs are intended to prevent all denials. Successful denial prevention programs will have the ability to appeal denials and should have a high overturn rate. If the review process that is part of the denial program has high inter-rater reliability, meaning that there is agreement on the outcomes of the reviews between the parties involved in the denial and appeal, and there is the ability to capture admissions that lead to proper reviews, then the overturn rate of denials should exceed 75%.

At the end of this chapter, the reader should be able to:

✔ Describe the appeals process

✔ Identify steps to ensure a high reversal rate

✔ List methods used to track denials

✔ Describe how to effectively use the tracked data

A 100% overturn rate is generally not achievable because you will find cases in which you agree with the review agency, be it the Centers for Medicare & Medicaid Services (CMS) or private payers, that the denial was appropriate. Agreeing with an admission denial can lead to increased revenue. A good example of improved reimbursement is a case in which the insurance company denies a short stay but approves an ambulatory to observation rate in which a percentage of charges will be paid. Short-stay diagnosis-related groups (DRG) or even a one- or two-day per

---

diem rate cannot begin to cover the charges for a procedure, and thus the payment for the ambulatory or observation rate at a percent of charges is greater than the other payment. If you agree to accept that payment, then your overturn rate cannot reach 100%, but the payment for ambulatory or observation is better than no payment at all.

Ensuring a High Reversal Rate

Reversal rates begin with the initial review process. Education of staff members about how to properly perform reviews is the foundation that must be in place to ensure a high reversal rate. Yearly review of staff competencies and ongoing case review with the utilization review (UR) committee are examples of best practices.

Data collection and analysis should be performed regularly and systematically to examine areas of weaknesses and opportunities. If there are doubts as to the UR process, a complete Plan-Do-Check-Act or Six Sigma project, whichever your organization uses for quality improvement strategies, should be undertaken to examine the reasons for a high denial rate and a low reversal rate. Examination of the top MS-DRGs service line, physician, and case manager (CM) denials should be quantified and qualified to understand the reasons for low performance. **Figure 5.1** comes from a Microsoft Access® database that is used to track denials. As stated in Chapter 3 under "Tracking Denials for Prevention," the ability to track denials efficiently will allow you to analyze the opportunities to target for marked improvement.

As soon as the areas of opportunities have been identified quality improvement initiatives can begin. Partnering with a quality department should be part of the improvement process. The quality department can assist in setting up tools to examine in depth the reasons behind the denials. Do not rely on anecdotal information; you must quantify and qualify the actionable areas. Quantifying them will allow you to track the time frame in which improvement activities began.

Figure 5.2 demonstrates the ability to track a process improvement activity in which there is a change in the number of denied days.

Understanding your weaknesses from a work flow perspective will also allow you to improve your ability to integrate best practices. Many improvement projects begin by completing a SWOT (strength, weakness, opportunity, and threat) analysis in which a cross-function team is assembled to discuss and brainstorm. **Figure 5.3** shows an example of a typical SWOT analysis.

From the information gathered you can establish a game plan for improvement in which the top three to five items are fully investigated and an improvement action plan is commenced.

Attention in the form of analysis and process improvement allows the CM performing reviews to improve his or her ability to reduce out-of-control areas. The front-end review process will ensure that patients are being admitted to the proper level of care.

FIGURE 5.1

Sample Microsoft Access Tracking Database

Type of denials:

#1 Admission,

#2 Lower level of care (inpatient to observation/ambulatory,

#3 Length of stay)

Date of Denial	Acct #	Admit Date	dx-DRG	Floor	Service	Physician	Payer	Type of Denial	Number of Days Denied
07-Feb-08		06-Feb-08	410	4SIR	MED		MVP	2	1
06-Mar-08		05-Mar-08	410	4SIR	GYN		MVP	2	1
24-Apr-08		02-Apr-08	410	4SIR	MED		MVP	2	1
02-May-08		30-Apr-08	410	4SIR	GYN		MVP	2	1
09-Jan-08		08-Jan-08		4SIR	MED		MVP	2	1
23-Jan-08		21-Jan-08	180	5PED	PED		MVP	2	1
17-Jan-08		17-Jan-08	298	5PED	PED		MVP	2	1
28-May-08		02-Nov-07	371	7NIR	OBS		MEDICAID	1	3
15-Jan-08		13-Apr-06	886	7SIR	ANP		MEDICAID	3	1
29-Feb-08		28-Feb-08	96	4NIR	GYN		MVP	2	1
15-Jan-08		22-Dec-07	832	6SIR	MED		AMERICHOICE	2	1

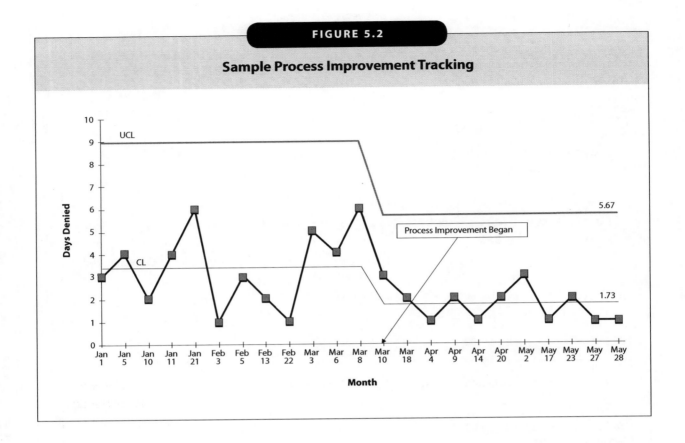

FIGURE 5.2

Sample Process Improvement Tracking

Prevent Denials and Win Appeals

FIGURE 5.3

Sample SWOT Analysis

Strengths
1. ECIN
2. Spectra-link
3. Huddles
4. Staff
5. Morning hospitalist rounds
6. Family meetings
7. Crisis intervention

Weaknesses
1. ECIN/IDX noninterface
2. Registration errors
3. Insurance Notifications
4. Lack of access to systems
5. Lack of access to Pisces
6. SW logging in to at least three different systems to obtain information
7. NCM logging in to at least seven different systems to obtain information
8. Volume of VM
9. Spectra-link interruptions
10. Printing of SW orders in ECIN/IDX
11. Incorrect consults
12. IDX orders only to SW with no NCM option
13. 45 minutes to organize day due to need to log into disparate systems, of which 20 minutes is all clerical work
14. Authorization follow-ups
15. Level II screens
16. Huddles
17. Chart reviews for DCP four to six hours daily, systems, chart location etc
18. Crisis intervention
19. Family meetings

Opportunities
1. ECIN/IDX interface
2. Insurance verification
3. Insurance card scanned but unable to access to view in HBF
4. Access to Pisces
5. SW IDX orders
6. Huddles
7. Access to systems
8. Lack of information for patients – DVDs, learning channel, etc

Threats
1. Registration entering incorrect status
2. Insurance verification
3. Lack of access to systems
4. Spectra-link
5. Huddles
6. Lack of time to meet new patients.

How to Write Proper Appeal Letters

The author has written and read many different appeal letters from various sources with a mixed success rate. Cookie-cutter templates are not effective. Detail in establishing medical necessity is the key. As stated in earlier chapters, the root of a denial is based on the perceived medical necessity of the admission or continued stay and professional services and treatment provided. To be effective, the letter must include details of the admission and the stay, as well as a description of the patient's acute care needs. The letter should be addressed to the individual or agent who will determine the outcome of the case.

All appeal letters should be structured in a manner that is consistent with presenting facts to a physician. The ultimate review agent is a physician with the knowledge and experience of the specialty for which the patient received treatment.

It is critical to verify where and to whom the letter should be sent because there is a limited time frame in which to appeal a denial. Sending your letter to the wrong division of an insurance company can waste valuable time and may even result in a permanent denial if you receive correspondence stating that the appeal was received after the deadline.

In the opening salutation, state to whom the letter is addressed. A typical salutation would be, "Dear Medical Reviewer," but if you know the name of the physician, address the letter to him or her by name.

The body of the letter should start with a recap of the denial. According to Employee Retirement Income Security Act (ERISA) regulations and most state public health or insurance laws, the denial appeal reviewer should be a different person than the initial reviewer, so the review will be de novo, meaning that to the reviewer this is a new case, and he or she is totally unfamiliar with this particular patient's story. Thus, it is best to recap the denial for the physician so he or she does not need to read the original or subsequent denial letters to understand the case.

The next section of your letter is where the appeal is won or lost; it is the battleground in which you pit your reasons for payment versus the reviewer's interpretation of the lack of medical necessity. At the end of this chapter is an example of a winning appeal letter. Outlining the medical needs of the patient as presented by the documentation in a logical, progressive nature in which you intersperse the criteria that were used to justify the admission is key to overturning the denial.

Other sections that should follow include evidence of standards of care, evidence of medical research that describes the care extended to the patient, and reiteration of any policy that the insurance company relied on and why it breached its own policy or a description of any plan in which the service provided is a covered service. Another section to consider, depending on the circumstances, is quoting the federal regulations of ERISA, which is described later in this chapter.

The end of the letter should wrap up your stance and state your expectations based on this de novo review.

Who Should Write Appeal Letters?

Appeal letters should be generated by an appeals nurse. Depending on the model, the appeals nurse might be part of the case management/utilization department, billing department, finance department, or even a separate appeals department. Some hospitals contract with companies that specialize in appeals, and they are responsible for generating the appeal letters, many times written at the behest of a physician. Whoever is charged with writing the letters should have knowledge of InterQual and a clinical background. Most facilities designate a nurse to write and sign the letter. The author has used a combination of methods, including his own wording, wording in collaboration with a physician advisor, the attending or a specialist, and sending joint letters—one written by the author and one by the physician. In some cases appeals may be referred to attorneys who handle the last level of appeal, sometimes at the administrative law judge level or even in a court of law.

ERISA

The federal government established ERISA in an effort to protect citizens' interest in their pension plans. The law was enacted in 1974 and has been ratified twice to add or extend health insurance and disability protection rights. The Consolidated Omnibus Budget Reconciliation Act of 1985 and the Health Insurance Portability and Accountability Act of 1996 were added to the regulation to provide further protections. Within the regulations is language that states that any insurance plan that is purchased through an employer gains protections of the act. The importance of this regulation is that it enables a healthcare facility to obtain information free of charge, under penalty of law.

The employer and review agent must provide the information, which includes how the decision to deny coverage is made, a copy of the patient's benefit plan (summary plan description), the information that was used to make the decision (including any internal policies), the name and specialty of the physician making the decision, and a full explanation of the denial, including the appeal process. The author has seen insurance companies provide an explanation of benefits (EOB) as the only communication of the denial in a line-item format, with a code stating that the denial was based on a lack of medical necessity, which is a violation of the ERISA statutes that preempt any state law in the interpretation of the plan.

Consider the following letter as a case study. Although patient names and any identifying information have been redacted, this is a real case in which a full reversal of the denial was achieved.

CASE STUDY

March 06, 2008

XYZ Insurance Company
Main Street
Anywhere, USA 12345

REGARDING:

MEMBER ID:

DOB:

DOS:

Dear Medical Reviewer:

Please accept this as an appeal in response to your October 20, 2007, adverse determination per the explanation of benefits denying the procedure of surgical implantation of a permanent percutaneous dual-lead dorsal column stimulator for your member. Your denial letter states that this service does not meet medical policy criteria. We respectfully disagree.

Ms. Doe was diagnosed with atypical complex regional pain syndrome (CRPS) of the abdomen complicated by atypical thoracic radiculopathy. She has a past surgical history of three cesarean sections and an exploratory laparotomy for endometriosis. She presented to the pain management specialist, Dr. Smith, with an examination resulting in dermatomal and nondermatomal patterns of pain from level T-6 through T-10/T-11. She also had skin manifestations to the abdomen in the form of blisters and ulcerations comparable with CRPS. She had trialed and failed multiple treatments consisting of multiple injections, neuro blocks, and hyperbaric oxygenation. She had undergone sympathetic blockades without long-term improvement. The medications Ms. Doe required for analgesia were Oxycodone 40 mg QID, Oxycontin 80 mg QID, Baclofen 20 mg QID, Celebrex 100 mg BID, Valium 30 mg QD, Methotrexate, and alternating doses of Tylenol and Ibuprofen and Ambien and Benadryl every night. Ms. Doe underwent a series of splenchnic nerve blocks with improvement of pain lasting five to seven days. On 06/25/2007 she underwent a surgical implantation of a percutaneous dual-lead dorsal column stimulator for trial to target the level of T5 through T8, which has primary control over the abdominal viscera and abdominal contents. She presented to ABC Hospital on 07/23/2007 for the procedure of fluoroscopic guided insertion of permanent electrodes of dorsal column stimulator and insertion of permanent subcutaneous extension with placement of a 16-channel rechargeable pulse generator. This permanent dorsal column

Prevent Denials and Win Appeals

stimulator was done as she reports a 50%–75% improvement in pain-level status postimplantation of the trial dorsal column stimulator. Per Dr. Smith's assessment, Ms. Doe also has improvement with almost total resolution of the percutaneous lesions and ulcerations of her abdomen since the trial procedure was performed on 06/25/2007.

The National Institute of Neurological Disorders and Stroke defines complex regional pain syndrome as a chronic pain condition with the key symptom of continuous, intense pain out of proportion to the severity of injury/invasive procedure, which gets worse rather than better over time (taking into account Ms. Doe's multiple abdominal surgeries). The institute describes typical features as dramatic changes in color and temperature of skin over the affected limb or body part (it does not describe affected areas as restricted to the extremities), accompanied by intense burning pain, skin sensitivity, sweating, and swelling (reference: *www.ninds.nih.gov*). Per the National Pain Foundation, the definition of pain can be "a disease in and of itself that needs to be diagnosed and managed as comprehensively as any other disease" (reference: *www.nationalpainfoundation.org*). In an article dedicated specifically to the diagnosis CRPS and evaluated by its peer review committee, the National Pain Foundation states, "The traditional thinking was that techniques designed to treat SMP, such as sympathetic blocks, were the only interventional strategies available. We now know that this is incorrect; however, as in many areas of medicine, new research and teaching has not yet caught up with many regional practice patterns." The article goes on to state that "spinal cord stimulation can be of considerable help in CRPS. SCS is generally first offered on a temporary basis and, if successful, is then used on a more permanent basis through surgery" (see enclosed article). An article written by Allen W. Burton, MD, Department of Anesthesiology and Pain Medicine at MD Anderson Cancer Center in Houston, a contributing author to the Reflex Sympathetic Dystrophy Association, states "Over time, much research and clinical experience has provided evidence that CRPS is a posttraumatic painful neurologic and inflammatory syndrome involving the somatosensory, sympathetic, and often the somatomotor systems" (see enclosed article). The article outlines the interventional pain treatment algorithm for CRPS encompassing a progression from minimally invasive therapies (i.e., sympathetic nerve blocks previously undergone by Ms. Doe without long-term success) progressing to more invasive therapies (i.e., neurostimulation). The article continues, stating, "existing data is positive in terms of pain reduction, quality of life, analgesic usage and function." In a study of 36 patients with advanced stages of CRPS (at least two years in duration), resulted pain levels averaged 53% better, which is "statistically significant." The article further reports a decrease in analgesic consumption in the majority of patients. The article further states, "The authors concluded that in the late stages of CRPS, neurostimulation (SCS or PNS) is a reasonable option when alternative therapies have failed," as is the case with Ms. Doe.

The explanation of benefits notes this claim is denied as it does not meet medical policy criteria. Per review of Policy Number: 7.01.51, Subject: Spinal Cord Stimulation, it is stated "Based upon our criteria and review of the peer-reviewed literature, spinal cord stimulation has been medically proven to be effective and, therefore, medically appropriate for treatment of patients with severe and chronic non-malignant pain of the trunk and limbs that is refractory to all other pain therapies." Ms. Doe does meet your policy guidelines inclusive of "the treatment is used only as a last resort. Other treatment modalities (pharmacological, surgical, psychological, or physical, if applicable) need to have been tried and failed or have been judged unsuitable or contraindicated, and demonstration of pain relief with a temporarily implanted electrode needs to precede permanent implantation. Patients are to be carefully screened, evaluated, and diagnosed by a multidisciplinary team prior to application of these therapies. All the facilities, equipment, and professional and support personnel required for the diagnosis, treatment, and follow-up of the patient need to be available." This policy had been last revised 04/19/2007, just prior to Ms. Doe undergoing these procedures.

Please note, we at ABC Hospital have not received a proper denial letter to date regarding this claim, as is our right under both the Public Health Law Article 4900 §4903 and the ERISA statute:

> §4903: Notice of an adverse determination made by a utilization review agent shall be in writing and must include:
> (a) The reasons for the determination including the clinical rationale, if any;
> (b) instructions on how to initiate standard and expedited appeals pursuant to section forty-nine hundred four and an external appeal pursuant to section forty-nine hundred fourteen of this article; and
> (c) notice of the availability, upon request of the enrollee, or the enrollee's designee, of the clinical review criteria relied upon to make such determination. Such notice shall also specify what, if any, additional necessary information must be provided to, or obtained by, the utilization review agent in order to render a decision on the appeal.

Per ERISA:
> When a plan administrator denies a claim for benefits in whole or in part, ERISA §503 and Labor Regulations Section 2560.503-1(f) require that a plan administrator must provide participant and beneficiary with written notice including all of the following information in a manner calculated to be understood by the claimant:
> 1. The specific reason for the denial;
> 2. Specific reference to the pertinent plan provisions on which the denial is based;
> 3. A description of any additional material or information necessary for the claimant to perfect the claim and an explanation of why such material is necessary; and
> 4. Appropriate information as to the steps to be taken if the participant or beneficiary wishes to submit his or her claim for review.

The ERISA Section 503(2) and the accompanying regulations require plans to provide an integral process for the appeal of any benefits claim denial. The review procedure must allow a claimant or his duly authorized representative to:

5. *Request a review upon written application to the plan,*
6. *Review pertinent documents, and*
7. *Submit issues and comments in writing.*

These requirements ensure that a claimant who appeals a denial to the plan administrator will be able to address the determinative issues and have a fair chance to present his case. A notice of benefits denial that does not provide the participant or beneficiary and the courts with a sufficiently precise understanding of the grounds for the denial to permit a realistic possibility of review will be considered inadequate.

(Employee Retirement Income Security Act of 1974; Rules and Regulations for Administration and Enforcement; Claims Procedure; Final Rule [11/21/2000] Volume 65, Number 225, pp. 70245-70271)

We expect that after a thorough review of the clinical data of this medical record a reversal of the denial will take place and authorization for the admission will be forthcoming. ABC Hospital does concur with XYZ Insurance Company that the main goal is for Ms. Doe to receive a quality and effective level of care. We do not feel this could have been established without the procedure, surgical implantation of a permanent percutaneous dual-lead dorsal column stimulator. If further information is needed, please feel free to contact me. We are also requesting a copy of all medical policies and criteria that your determination is based on, along with the credentials of the medical reviewer rendering this medical necessity review as is our right under the Public Health Law Article 4900 §4903.

Summary

Building a case for the reversal of a denial should be individualized to a patient's circumstance. As stated earlier, cookie-cutter templates achieve little success. Creating excellent, winning appeal letters takes a dedicated individual who understands clinical information and can use research to obtain the necessary information that will lead to reversals. Establishing a trend with insurance companies will also lead to better relationships, as dialogues should commence once you demonstrate your ability to consistently overturn denials.

Reporting

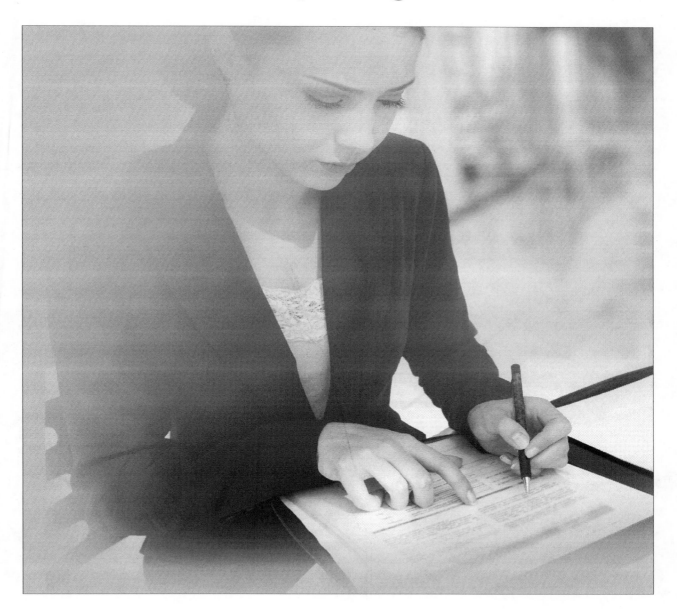

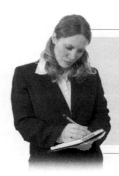

Reporting

CHAPTER 6

The Value of Reporting Denial Data

Reporting denial data is an important function of any denial and appeals process for many reasons, including the justification of time staff members spend in bringing the process to fruition, showing the return on investment of added staff or the expense of appealing denials, and justifying changes to contractual agreements. It is also useful for setting monthly meetings with private payers to discuss and overturn denials.

Capturing the actual work being done and trending reports will allow further analysis that can lead to process improvement; building relationships with finance, the business office, and the medical staff; and streamlining the revenue cycle. Data in the healthcare environment are used to create new methods that lead to improved revenue streams. The finance department may not view case management departments as an integral function of the revenue stream but rather as an adjunct to capturing reimbursement. When the reimbursement process does not work efficiently, fingers often point to case management; when the process goes well, the department is seldom given kudos. Knowing what to report and how to report it will enable case management and utilization departments to prove that the investment of

time and resources is supporting improved revenue streams. This chapter will address how to capture and report data regardless of the budget set aside for information technology to assist the case management or utilization department. Included are examples from a simple database that was created using Microsoft Access but that can be reproduced using other reporting tool software programs or an Excel spreadsheet.

LEARNING OBJECTIVES

At the end of this chapter, the reader should be able to:

✔ Identify which data to report

✔ Determine how to organize data for reporting

✔ Determine to whom the data should be reported

✔ List tools used to report the data

✔ Relate the importance of generating appropriate reports

What to Report

Recognizing what to report is just as important as knowing to whom to report or which data to capture. The first step is to understand how denials occur. Reading and tracking the denials by type in whichever code, or category is set up is a key process that must be agreed on by the stakeholders to elicit proper responses to the data. In the author's experience, being able to report data that can be easily understood by the layperson will facilitate communication concerning the processes that require improvement. **Figures 6.1–6.4** are some examples of data that can and should be reported monthly. Display the data in an easily understood format so that it will lead to open discussion of the issues that resulted in denials.

Figure 6.1 is an example of a quarterly report on denial by payer source.

Figure 6.2 is an example of denials by service line for a quarter.

Figure 6.3 is an example of denials by type for a quarter.

Figure 6.4 delineates the denials that occurred during a quarter by service line from an inpatient status to an observation level of care.

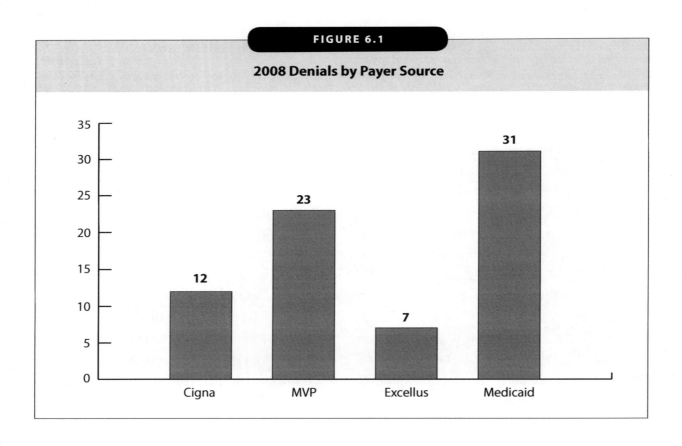

FIGURE 6.1

2008 Denials by Payer Source

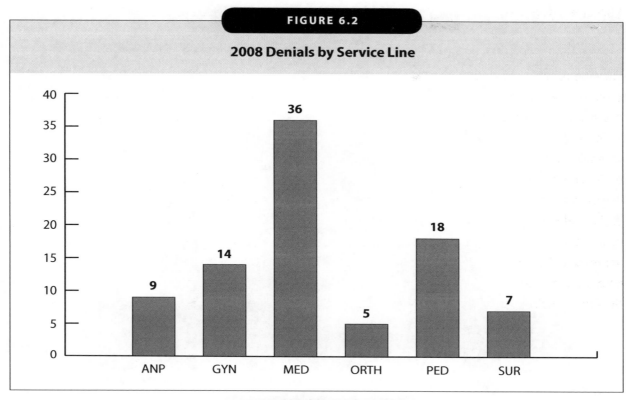

FIGURE 6.2

2008 Denials by Service Line

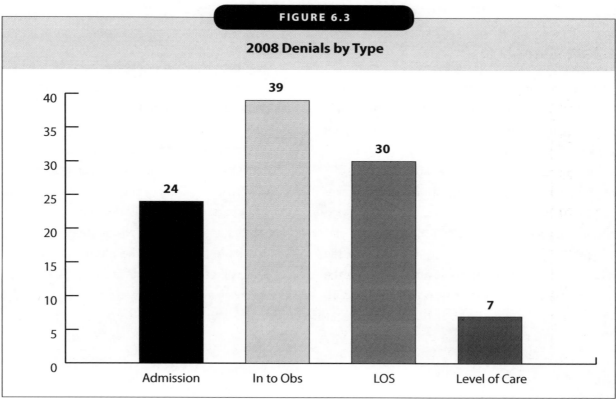

FIGURE 6.3

2008 Denials by Type

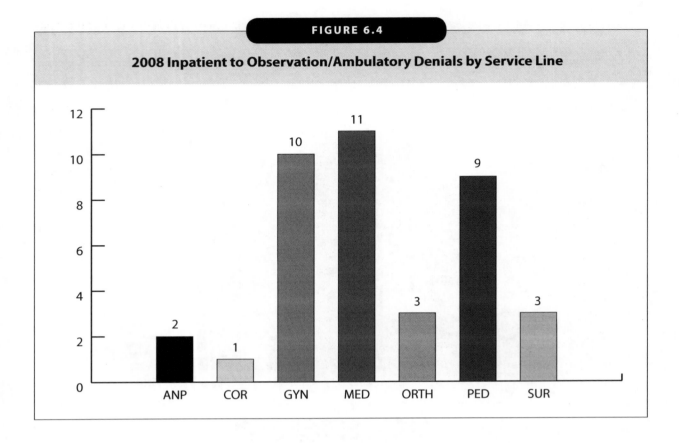

FIGURE 6.4

2008 Inpatient to Observation/Ambulatory Denials by Service Line

Who to Report to

Most healthcare organizations have a reporting structure that requires case management to provide information on its performance to the overall hospital leadership, such as the CEO, CMO, CNO, and the CFO. If those requirements include denials and appeals, the information should be shared with the proper stakeholders. However, in some organizations, identifying the stakeholders can be challenging. To be sure that the proper committees and individuals receive the information that will be reviewed and acted upon, the leadership team should design reports that will ensure

that the data reported meets the needs of the individuals that can affect the process of denials and appeals and increase compliance.

Denial prevention begins up front with the emergency, patient access, and outpatient departments—in other words, the points of entry. The reports should reach key personnel who make decisions about admission status and who have power over the correct admission process. Provide the information in a manner that will be easily assimilated and disseminated. The following examples show information provided in a manner that can influence transformational change and displayed in a format that will allow personnel to pinpoint changes to processes.

Figure 6.5 displays information in a control chart, also known as a run chart, which demonstrates the total denial rate. Information can be pointed to that speaks to the process changes that occurred to decrease the denial rate. In this example, in October 2005, the ED case management program began to review cases prior to admission. In March 2006, caseload balancing of case manager to patient was decreased to a 1:20 ratio along with a complex discharge facilitator.

Figure 6.6 shows the overall overturn rate. Positive changes can be attributed to increases in staff ratios, ED case management reviews, and a change in physician documentation on the necessity of admissions. By the first quarter of 2009, the reversal rate increased to more than 70%.

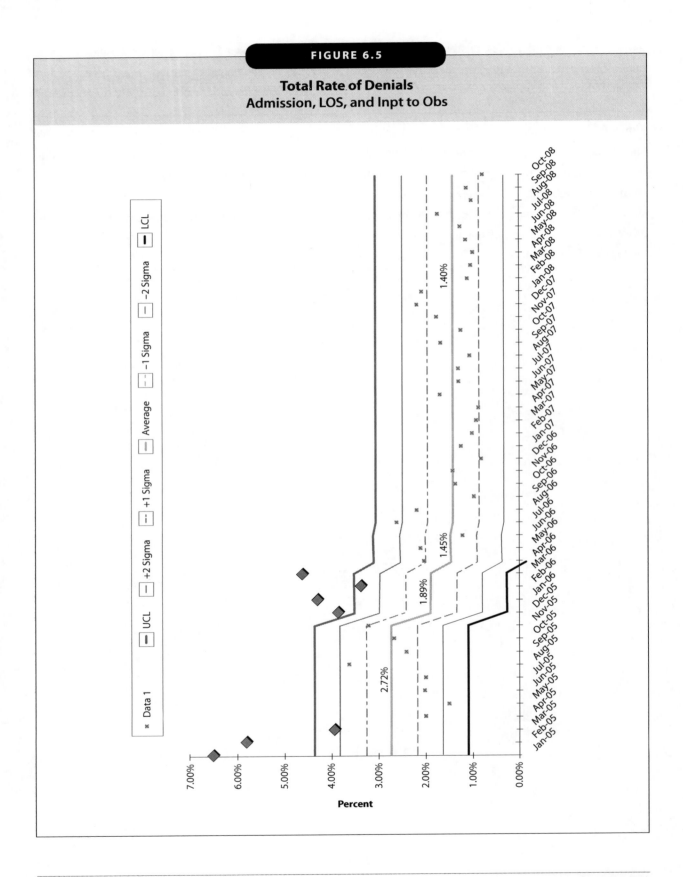

FIGURE 6.5

Total Rate of Denials
Admission, LOS, and Inpt to Obs

Prevent Denials and Win Appeals

FIGURE 6.6

Monthly Denial Reversal Rate

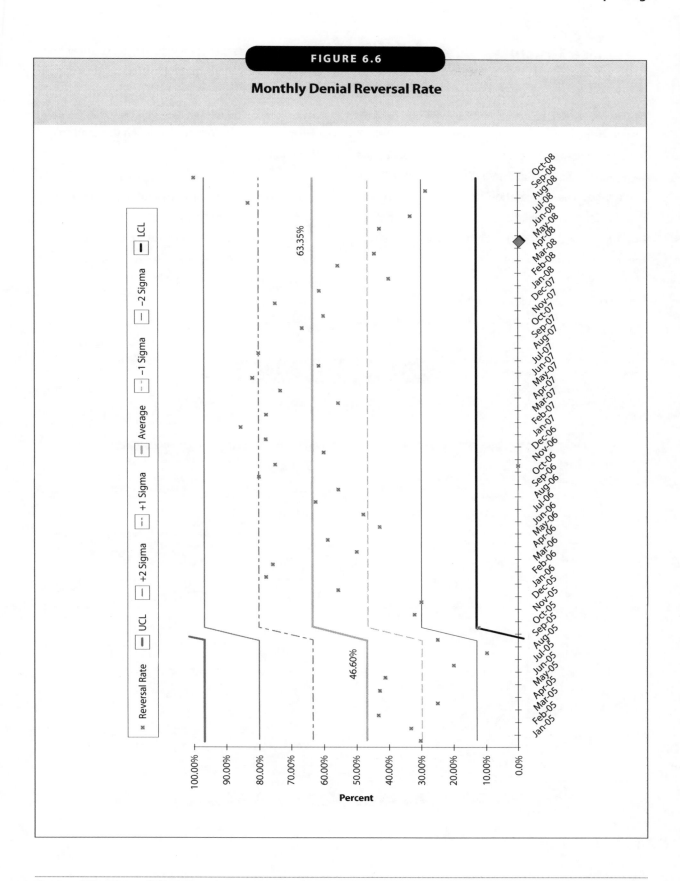

Database Structure

As previously stated, creating a database can be as simple as making an Excel® spreadsheet and as complex as using a software suite. Other simple solutions include a Microsoft Access database. The following two figures show what the author created to track and analyze the information that led to the preceding charts. Most facilities have experts in information technology who can create simple, cost-effective reporting mechanisms.

Figure 6.7 is an example of a simple Microsoft Access database that was created in a few hours but has all of the elements necessary to generate meaningful reports such as those that have been displayed in this chapter, based on the captured data. From this database, reports and queries can be created and used to further drill down data that can and will lead to positive changes.

Figure 6.8 is an example of a pivot table created from the information in the preceding database. Pivot tables allow users to analyze data in a variety of ways and manipulate the information without the need to compute information manually.

FIGURE 6.7

Database Sample (Microsoft Office)

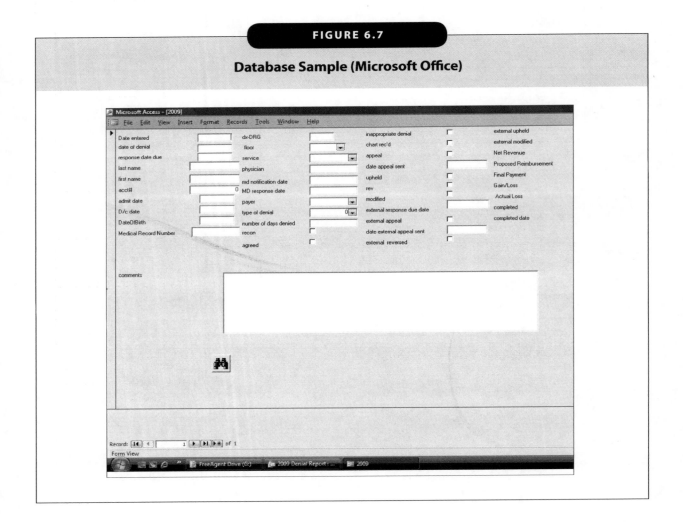

FIGURE 6.8

Pivot Table Example

Payer	Data	Total
AETNA	Sum of actual loss	0
	Sum of gain\loss	1848.21
ANTHEM	Sum of actual loss	0
	Sum of gain\loss	7403.69
BC	Sum of actual loss	0
	Sum of gain\loss	3827.52
CIGNA	Sum of actual loss	-7905.8
	Sum of gain\loss	10260.05
EMPIRE	Sum of actual loss	-575.37
	Sum of gain\loss	8533.06
EXCELLUS	Sum of actual loss	-34738.36
	Sum of gain\loss	-13895.33
FIDELIS	Sum of actual loss	0
	Sum of gain\loss	4998.33
GHI	Sum of actual loss	0
	Sum of gain\loss	5403.77
MEDICAID	Sum of actual loss	-6188.94
	Sum of gain\loss	50171.62
MVP	Sum of actual loss	-19897.63
	Sum of gain\loss	-6709.29
OTHER	Sum of actual loss	0
	Sum of gain\loss	16388.91
TOUCHSTONE	Sum of actual loss	0
	Sum of gain\loss	1044.36
UNITED HEALTH CARE	Sum of actual loss	-1907.69
	Sum of gain\loss	10584.71
Total Sum of actual loss		**-71213.79**
Total Sum of gain\loss		**99859.61**

Summary

Reporting meaningful information to proper stake-holders can lead to positive transformational changes that will allow case management and utilization departments to demonstrate their return on investment. Displaying information that is consistent with proven outcomes by quality improvement efforts also helps legitimize these departments' roles as a consistent and proven methodology. The medical staff is accustomed to seeing data reported in a manner that displays quality standards. The use of control/run charts will help prompt discussions about improvement initiatives that can be tracked and measured.

All quality improvement processes should begin with data management and the creation of a tracking tool that can use data to generate reports that contain and validate action items.

Contracting

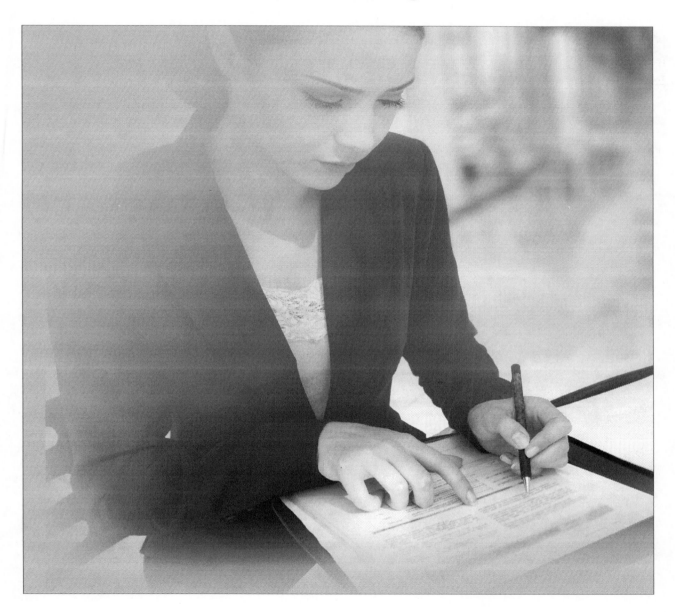

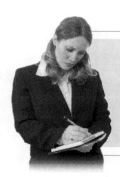

Contracting

Providing a Reimbursement Methodology

Contracts or agreements between a hospital and a private insurance company, commonly referred to as a payer or managed care organization are primarily designed to provide a reimbursement methodology that is beneficial for both parties. An agreement creates a contractual relationship that permits a hospital to have access to the insurance network, which includes patients, physicians, and third-party sources such as nursing homes, durable medical equipment vendors, home health agencies, and other entities that contract with the insurance company. This network access is beneficial for the patient and the hospital, as it creates an avenue to share in discounted pricing and to take advantage of the insurance company's relationships by moving patients to the most appropriate level of care when needed. The insurance company benefits because it can reduce the cost of care in a negotiated payment rate that, in most cases, is less than usual and customary charges. Being able to reduce cost allows the insurance companies to provide coverage for more enrollees.

Agreements have many business and binding legal features that create a framework for a working relationship. Within most provider agreements, there is language that delineates medical necessity review.

The contractual agreement between the hospital and the insurance company differs from a summary plan description (SPD) in that the SPD is intended to be the written plan to provide coverage for the beneficiary, and the provider agreement specifies the method of conducting business between the hospital and the insurance company. Within the body of the contract, medical necessity as well as the review and appeals processes are defined. Careful attention should be paid to the wording of the agreement to ensure compliance with federal and state regulatory and insurance laws. Incorporating language that follows these regulations and laws is necessary to protect review and appeals rights of the hospital.

Other areas for consideration in a contract are sections discussing reimbursement in terms of level of care. For example, if a facility has only two levels of neonatal intensive care, the agreement should only contain reimbursement rates for those two levels. This avoids future debate over which level the baby was in and at what reimbursement rate. Another example is rates for skilled nursing care. If the hospital does not have a skilled nursing unit or swing beds (i.e., unoccupied acute care beds used as skilled level of care for patients when other skilled care beds are not available), having a rate for a lower level of care is not necessary. In fact, if there is a skilled nursing level of care reimbursement rate in a hospital contract, it may open the door for level of care denials. This chapter will provide information on how to interpret the language in the contract and how to strategize with the contracting personnel within your facility to create a more robust agreement.

How to Incorporate Denial Prevention into Hospital and Payer Agreements/Contracts

Most hospitals have a corporate-level person or persons with the primary responsibility of writing contracts. Contracts are written for precise lengths of time, also known as a term of agreement. When a contract term expires, it is customary to review the contract and propose appropriate changes that are beneficial to both parties. Financial elements of the contract are worked out with the finance department. However, case management should be involved in reviewing the language of the contract as it pertains to the medical review and appeals processes. It may also participate in negotiating the rate for the different levels of care that exist in the hospital.

At times, the parties cannot agree on the precise language, and counsel must be consulted to determine the proper format. From a case management perspective, what is needed are clear concepts that outline definitions that will ensure compliance with regulations and processes and create a fair and balanced approach to determine medical necessity. As stated throughout this book, reimbursement is predicated on providing care that is medically necessary. It is essential to have a defined process for dispute resolution that is consistent with regulations and protects each beneficiary's rights and, thus, the hospital's rights. The scope and purpose of agreed-upon dispute resolution language is to provide a forum that will minimize cost expenditures for both parties. If an appeal reaches the level of the courts, the associated costs, and the opportunity to have a positive return on investment, may be insufficient to proceed. If the costs to take an appeal to court exceed the potential reimbursement, a decision must be made as to whether it is reasonable to pursue the denial. Having an agreeable, binding relationship creates a manageable process to appeal any denial and establishes a framework of understanding for the review process. The review process outlined in most agreements includes precertification, concurrent, and retrospective reviews. The agreements will contain language on how the process of review is conducted and who will conduct it. Most case management or utilization review departments do not get involved in prehospital reviews, as they are used mostly for elective surgeries. The areas that most affect case management are the initial, concurrent, and retrospective review processes. Following is an example of contract language that discusses the concurrent review process, as well as collaborative agreements for discharge planning:

1. The goal of the concurrent review is to determine whether inpatient hospital services are medically necessary covered services for a member. Case management services may include but are not limited to authorization and arrangement of posthospital services such as skilled nursing care, durable medical equipment, and outpatient services such as physical therapy, respiratory therapy, or phlebotomy. Insurance company reviewers, referred to as payer-based case managers, collaborate with the hospital discharge planner to identify and obtain services. Selection of postacute service providers is accomplished by hospital staff members based on payer contractual arrangements with those providers.

2. If the payer approves inpatient hospital services following concurrent review, the payer shall not retrospectively deny such services as not medically necessary unless the information upon which the payer relied in making its determination was materially misrepresented.

3. The payer shall use criteria such as InterQual or Milliman Care Guidelines to determine medical necessity, level of care, and admission status.

4. If a member's admission does not meet criteria for acute care, the payer-based reviewer such as case manager, will contact the hospital-based case manager, or the patient's physician to discuss the patient's clinical criteria to determine whether there is additional information that is not documented in the medical record. Assuming no change in determination, the case will then be referred for review by The Insurance Company medical director and, when possible, the hospital chief medical officer or his or her designee.

5. If there is insufficient information provided to justify an acute inpatient stay for the member, The Insurance Company shall issue a concurrent denial. If The Insurance Company denies hospital services, The Insurance Company will issue a denial in accordance with company protocol and state and federal law. The Insurance Company reviewer will also notify the member's attending physician and the hospital appeal coordinator via telephone and in writing.

6. The Insurance Company reviewers will work collaboratively with the hospital

utilization management department personnel, discharge planning staff, and the ancillary hospital services department personnel to assist with discharge planning needs for the member.

By adding structure within the agreement, ambiguity about the review and appeal process is eliminated and each party better understands its role. The sample language included here is from an actual hospital agreement that came about after years of an adversarial relationship. Due to a poorly worded contract that included rates for skilled nursing and four levels of NICU care, which didn't exist at the hospital, the insurance company was subject to state review for its denial processes. This is a situation that can be avoided by carefully worded contracts.

Language to Include in the Agreement

Other language that should be included in the contract will vary from state to state depending on the dispute resolution that is agreed upon and the availability of a third-party binding arbitrator. Regulations or laws that affect the dispute resolution process do not necessarily need to be included but add weight to the process that both parties need to follow. The contract language should also contain timelines to receive and send denials and appeals as required by federal ERISA laws and or state laws. For example, the following language is from a New York state contract and can be used as a template to create an agreement that will outline the process and bind the parties to a dispute resolution process.

SAMPLE TEMPLATE

A. In order to provide a single forum for all disputes that may arise under this Agreement with respect to specific claims, disputes between Health Plan and Hospital (involving only members who are not covered by Medicare or Medicaid) pertaining to the following types of matters shall be resolved under the process set forth in this Section only. In order to obtain the benefit of the single forum for all disputes, Hospital expects to utilize this one comprehensive forum. Health Plan's determination on any of the following matters need not be in the form of a written denial letter before this process may be initiated, and a rejected claims statement or a claims adjustment shall be a sufficient basis for initiating the process. Further, "approval" of a level of care different from the level of care Hospital believes is appropriate shall be a sufficient basis for initiating the process. Notwithstanding the above, Hospital has the option to utilize this one comprehensive forum or the external review process with respect to disputes reviewable at Hospital's request under §4910 of the New York Public Health Law or §4910 of the New York Insurance Law. Nothing in this Section is intended, nor shall it be construed, as precluding Hospital from serving as an authorized representative of a claimant, as that term is used in Section 2560.503-1 of Title 29 of the *Code of Federal Regulations,* and pursuing all actions and rights as provided for such claimants under an employee benefits plan pursuant to federal law. Either Health Plan can request this process or Hospital can request this process. The types of matters covered by this procedure include:

i. Determinations by Health Plan with respect to precertification or hospital inpatient care services which are contrary to the determination which Hospital believes should have been made, including without limitation, the denial of coverage, the denial of precertification, or the granted precertification at a level of care which is lower than the level of care requested by Hospital admitting physician.

ii. Retrospective determinations relating to medical necessity, level of care, or DRG assignment.

iii. Emergency service and ambulatory care service denials or "downcoding" or "upcoding" ("approval" of a level of care different from the level of care Hospital believes appropriate).

iv. Disputes regarding the correctness or completeness of records or information.

v. Disputes seeking adjustment of any payments or adjustments which have been calculated by relying on any incorrect or incomplete records or information.

vi. Disputes arising out of contract compliance audits (based on sampling methodology) if level of care is an integral component of the issues raised, but the sampling methodology shall not be subject to this Section.

vii. Such other disputes as the parties mutually agree in writing to make subject to the terms of this Section.

The foregoing notwithstanding, nothing herein shall be deemed to authorize or require the disclosure of personally identifiable patient information or information related to other individual healthcare providers or Health Plan's proprietary data collection systems, software, or quality assurance or utilization review methodologies.

B. Procedure. Hospital must request the appeal by giving notice to Health Plan in writing, including the basis for the appeal, within thirty (30) days after the notification by Health Plan to Hospital of Health Plan's determination. The time frame for appeal will begin once Hospital receives the determination. In situations in which Hospital receives a denied remittance/letter, the time frame will begin as of the date Hospital receives the denied remittance/letter, and Hospital agrees to submit the denied remittance/letter with the appeal. This appeal process does not replace the existing retrospective review process, but it does apply to any disputes arising out of such retrospective review process. Each appeal shall proceed through three levels, unless the parties otherwise agree in writing. An agreement to vary the three-level appeal process in one case shall not be deemed an agreement to vary the three-level appeal process in any other case.

   i. Level I: Health Plan's staff shall review the matter and conclude that review within thirty (30) days after Health Plan receives notice of Hospital's appeal. If Hospital still does not agree with Health Plan's decision, Hospital may within one hundred eighty days (180) after receiving the Level I decision, notify Health Plan of Hospital's request for a Level II appeal.

   ii. Level II: A request for a second level appeal will be reviewed by Health Plan's medical director and will be concluded within thirty (30) days after Health Plan receives Hospital's request for a Level II appeal. The foregoing notwithstanding, at any point during the review process Hospital staff (most frequently registered nurses, medical director, attending/consulting physicians) may initiate dialogue with Health Plan's medical director or utilization review staff regarding medical necessity (including level of care) decisions, but Hospital must still follow the appeal process as set forth in this Section. If Hospital still does not agree with the decision of Health Plan's medical director, Hospital may, when applicable, request a Level III appeal within thirty (30) days after receiving such decision.

   iii. Level III: The third level of appeals will be submitted to the following designated Dispute Resolution Agency ("DRA"):

NY State Review Service

120 Main Street

Somewhere, NY 11002

Whenever Hospital submits a dispute to the DRA, Hospital shall simultaneously provide Health Plan with a copy of such dispute resolution request, including all of the materials which accompanied that request. Hospital shall also provide Health Plan with any additional materials thereafter supplied to the DRA. Similarly, Health Plan shall provide Hospital with copies of all materials Health Plan submits to the DRA. All reviews by the DRA shall be conducted in accordance with the terms of Title 10 of the *New York State Code of Rules and Regulations*, §86-1.83 as filed on March 19, 1991, and amended on April 1, 1994, and July 13, 1994, notwithstanding the expiration of these provisions on December 31, 1996, as applicable to Health Plan, provided, however, that in reviewing such disputes, the DRA shall use InterQual or another nationally recognized criteria, as such criteria may have been modified by locally adopted community standards. The types of disputes that may be submitted for review shall be strictly limited to those described in this Section. The fee for a dispute resolution is to be paid initially by the requesting party and is nonrefundable. In the event the party which initially paid this fee prevails in the dispute, the non-requesting party shall reimburse the requesting party for the fee.

    iv. The parties acknowledge that the Commissioner of Health is not bound by arbitration or mediation decisions. Arbitration or mediation shall occur within New York state, and the Commissioner of Health will be given notice of all issues going to arbitration or mediation, and copies of all decisions.

C. Obligations in Connection with Dispute Resolution. In addition to the hold harmless and no balance billing provisions of this Agreement, if Health Plan makes a determination with respect to precertification or hospital inpatient care services that is contrary to the determination which Hospital believes should have been made, including and, without limitation, the denial of precertification or the granted precertification at a level of care that is lower than the level of care agreed to by Health Plan and Hospital admitting physician, then:

    i. Hospital shall not advise the member that the specific services or the suggested level of care are noncovered, or that the member will be liable for the cost of the service or the difference in cost between the cost of the level of care requested by Hospital admitting physician and the level of care approved by Health Plan's case manager;

    ii. Hospital shall not bill, charge, collect a deposit from, seek compensation, remuneration or reimbursement from, or have any recourse against the member or person (other than Health Plan) acting on his/her/their behalf, for the services rendered;

    iii. Hospital shall continue to be solely responsible for providing care in a manner consistent with its own sound medical judgment and practice, notwithstanding Health Plan's decision. However, notwithstanding the foregoing, nothing in this Section is intended nor shall it be construed as requiring Hospital to provide services to members if the Hospital is not otherwise legally obligated to do so if the Hospital determines, based upon the precertification decision of the Health Plan, that it cannot provide such services in light of Health Plan's reimbursement decision and as precluding the Hospital from informing the member of the reason it is declining to provide such services;

    iv. The decision by Health Plan will be appealable under this Section; the DRA is expressly authorized to participate in the resolution of such an appeal in accordance with the provisions of this Section if so requested by either party;

    v. Hospital shall accept as its full compensation, and Health Plan shall pay, the amount determined to be due by the appeal process; and

    vi. Prior determinations by Health Plan or acceptance by Hospital of Health Plan's prior determination concerning the level of care approved with respect to a type of medical condition shall not be deemed to indicate Health Plan's decision or acceptance by Hospital of Health Plan's decision, on future requests for precertification.

Note that in the language there is a hold harmless clause to not bill the member for a medical necessity denial regardless of the outcome. The hospital is acting on the beneficiary's behalf when appealing a denial and thus to bill the patient for an error in judgment in admitting him or her is not consistent with good medical practice. However, this is not to say that if a member presents an invalid insurance card or has had his or her coverage terminated the hospital should not bill the patient. In essence, the patient then becomes a self-pay patient. The hospital should bill the patient, and the denial should not be counted in the total denial rate.

Case management should engage the department responsible for writing contracts with payers and participate in the contracting process to review and provide guidance about the appeals process. It is within the contracting phase that many future denials can be prevented. Case management can demonstrate denial reduction and thus show the value of changes to contract language. This is a unique opportunity to be involved in the quality improvement process. Measure and document the denial rates prior to the changes recommended in contract language and compare them to the rates post changes. Remember that to have a high level of confidence in the data, you must have enough data points to prove any trend is valid. Tracking and trending denial rates over time with contract language points indicated is a good way to show improvement. For example: fiscal year (FY) 2006 had 100 denials. Case management was involved in contract language modifications for FY 2007. Denials for 2007 dropped to 50. Other factors may have contributed to the drop, but case management involvement in the contract process was one of the key factors.

Consent Form Language

To appeal a denial, the hospital must obtain the consent or agreement from the member beneficiary. Federal regulations within ERISA state the following:

> *The claims procedures do not preclude an authorized representative of a claimant from acting on behalf of such claimant in pursuing a benefit claim or appeal of an adverse benefit determination. Nevertheless, a plan may establish reasonable procedures for determining whether an individual has been authorized to act on behalf of a claimant (ERISA §2560.503-1 (b) (4) Federal Register, Vol. 65, No. 225, Tuesday, November 21, 2000, Rules and Regulations, p. 70266).*

Most interpretations of this regulation provide that an assignment of benefits is sufficient to meet the requirement. The assignment of benefits is done at the time the member is admitted to the hospital and states that the hospital can bill the member's payer for services. Some insurance companies and external review agencies require further consent to allow the hospital to appeal on behalf of the beneficiary. Putting appeal rights language in the consent for treatment is an effective mechanism to ensure that the hospital has obtained the right to appeal. The challenge in this approach is ensuring that the patient's or the patient's representative has actually signed the consent form. A process should be established to obtain the signature prior to the patient leaving the hospital. Having the consent prior to the patient leaving is easier than writing to a patient to obtain consent. Patients may not respond, they may have moved, or they may have life-changing events that prevent them from completing the assignment of benefits form after discharge.

The following is an example of consent language that will allow any facility to act on behalf of the beneficiary to pursue an appeal and that meets the regulation as stated above:

> *I understand that there will be medical expenses associated with the care I receive from Hospital. In consideration of these medical expenses, I, the undersigned, to the extent I have insurance or employee health care benefits coverage, hereby assign and convey directly to Hospital all medical benefits and insurance reimbursement, if any, otherwise payable to me for services rendered by Hospital and its affiliated doctors and other providers. In addition, I assign such medical benefits payable for physician services to the physicians furnishing such services. I understand that I am financially responsible for all charges (regardless of any applicable insurance or benefit payments, if any). I hereby authorize any plan administrator or fiduciary, insurer, and my attorney to release to Hospital any and all health plan documents, insurance policies, and settlement information upon written request from Hospital to claim such medical benefits, reimbursement, or any applicable remedies. I authorize the use of this signature on all my insurance and employee health benefits claim submissions.*

> *I hereby convey to Hospital, to the fullest extent allowed by law and under any applicable insurance policies and employee health plan, any claim, the right to bring a claim, or other rights I may have under such insurance or employee health plan for medical expenses related to the care I received from Hospital and, to the extent allowable by law, to claim such medical benefits, insurance reimbursement, and any applicable remedies. Further, in response to a reasonable request by Hospital, I agree to cooperate with Hospital in any attempts by Hospital to bring a claim or assert a right against my insurers or employee health plan, including, if necessary, to bring suit with Hospital against such insurers or employee health plan in my name but at Hospital's expense.*

The consent language also authorizes the facility to request an SPD and or any other relevant information in relation of the pursuit of payment from the insurance company.

Joint Resolution Process

The joint resolution process is another example of a tool to improve collaboration and make the denial appeal process more stable and efficient. For example, the insurance company mentioned in the beginning of the chapter that was reviewed by the state proposed that the hospital enjoin in a joint dispute resolution process. The process became part of the agreement and has led to positive outcomes for both parties. Being able to meet and discuss denials provided a venue for understanding each other's definition of medical necessity and assisted in decreasing the overall denial rate. The following is the language that was placed in the agreement with that particular insurance company:

The purpose of this joint dispute resolution process is to promote communication and a better understanding of the utilization services and patterns for both Hospital and the Company, provide a collaborative setting to resolve disagreements, and reduce administrative burden of the formal two step appeal process. The Company and Hospital will use the outcomes of this reconsideration process to improve utilization practices. In a cooperative effort, the Company and Hospital will form a joint dispute resolution group consisting of one physician medical director from the Hospital and one physician medical director from the Company. Individuals, who are their entities representatives, shall consistently attend the meetings. Only nonphysician case management staff members from the Company and Hospital may attend the meetings to support the process.

The group will meet monthly at a mutually agreed upon location to review all cases submitted to the Company for reconsideration by the Hospital, within sixty (60) days of the date the Hospital receives the adverse determination notice from the Company. The group shall determine operating protocol to ensure an efficient and effective discussion and dispute resolution process. Should the Hospital not file its request for review through the joint dispute resolution process within the time frames defined in the paragraph, the Hospital may use the usual process as defined by the Company's protocols.

If, after review of cases, discussion, and reconsideration, the medical directors of the Company and Hospital agree on the resolution of the disputed case, both parties agree to honor the decision, and the Company's staff will immediately implement the decision via the Company's claim payment system.

If the Company's and Hospital's medical directors do not agree, the Hospital may submit the case for appeal through the usual established process set forth in the Company protocol.

Summary

Contracting and consent language are additional weapons in the arsenal to prevent denials and win appeals. The language of the contract can create beneficial processes that can lead to increased collaboration. Case managers, with frontline and day-to-day experience in how medical necessity is applied to a member's admission and continued stay, are key players in writing contract language. By becoming an active part of the contracting process, the appeal process will become more organized because there will be fewer denials based on ambiguous processes.

Recovery Audit Contractors

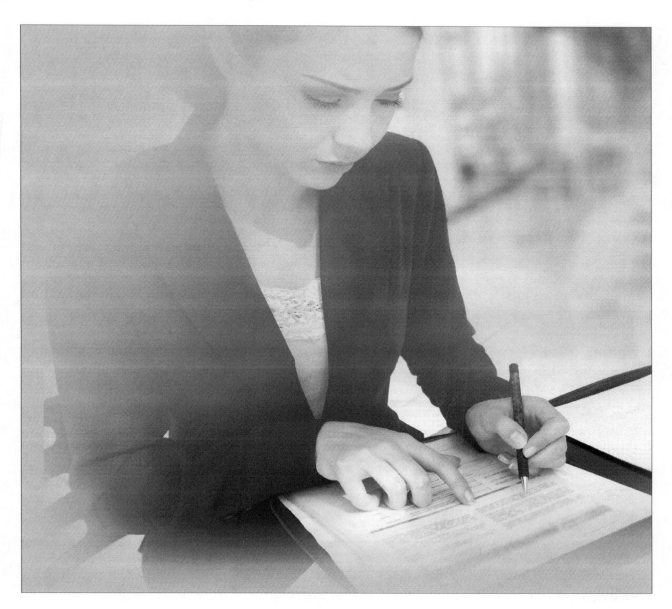

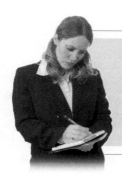

Recovery Audit Contractors

CHAPTER 8

The Purpose Behind RAC

In Section 306 of the Medicare Prescription Drug, Improvement and Modernization Act of 2003, Congress directed the U.S. Department of Health and Human Services to conduct a three-year demonstration using recovery audit contractors, now referred to simply as RACs, to detect and correct improper payments, both overpayments and underpayments, in the Medicare fee-for-service (FFS) program. Congress gave the Centers for Medicare & Medicaid Services (CMS) the authority to pay each RAC on a contingency fee basis, which is a percentage of the improper payments corrected by the RACs.

CMS designed the RAC program to:

1. Detect and correct past improper payments in the Medicare FFS program.

2. Provide information to CMS and Medicare contractors that could help protect the Medicare Trust Funds by preventing future improper payments, thereby lowering the Medicare FFS claims payment error rate.

Congress made the RAC program permanent when it enacted the Tax Relief and Health Care Act of 2006, which directs CMS to expand a permanent

At the end of the chapter, the reader should be able to:

✔ Describe the genesis of the Recovery Audit Contractor (RAC) program

✔ Implement strategies to prevent RAC denials

✔ Appeal a RAC denial

RAC program to all 50 states by 2010. CMS intended to implement the permanent RAC program in phases beginning in October 2008. As of March 27, 2008, RACs succeeded in correcting more than $1.03 billion in Medicare improper payments. Approximately 96% ($992.7 million) of the improper payments were overpayments that were recouped from providers, whereas the remaining 4% ($37.8 million) were underpayments repaid to providers. The Medicare Secondary Payer RACs collected fewer overpayments

($12.7 million) than the claim RACs ($980 million). RACs are expected to look back up to three years, starting with October 1, 2007, focusing on short stays (one and three days) for medical necessity, incorrectly coded claims, and other payment errors such as old fee schedules.

The permanent RAC program uses automated proprietary software programs with decision algorithms to identify potential payment errors. The process to find a potential error has two incremental methods:

- **Automated review:** Passes review or demand letter

- **Complex review:** Requests a copy of medical record

The first is a screen in which the claim is screened automatically to detect payment errors. In the second method, known as a complex review, the RAC requests a copy of the patient's medical record review by one of the RAC claims reviewers. RAC reviewers are highly trained staff members: coders, nurses, or physicians.

Once the information is received and reviewed, the RAC will notify the facility of its findings, which could include one of three types of notices:

- No errors were found

- an informational letter with notification that an overpayment occurred

- an underpayment was discovered and the hospital is entitled to further payment

Understanding the risk areas is key to developing strategies to prevent a RAC denial. The RAC appeal process is no different from any other denial prevention program. The program should begin with a systematic review based on the admissions known to most commonly be denied. Reviewing medical records will demonstrate the weaknesses and strengths of the organization that will illuminate previously unknown areas of opportunities.

How to Prevent Losses to RAC via Denial Prevention

As stated in the introduction to this chapter, prevention starts with the discovery of the areas of strengths or weaknesses. Medicare, until 2009, provided a PEPPER report, which gave hospitals information highlighting overall performance compared to other hospitals in the state. The insight provided by the report outlined the areas on which the RAC would focus. Case management or utilization departments should work with finance and health information management departments to re-create a report based on the elements of the PEPPER report to internally monitor the areas that may be of concern. Knowing which diagnoses or types of stays are problematic (e.g., one-day, three-day, or skilled nursing facility) will enable you to concentrate your efforts to prevent denials. If 100% review of all admissions is not achievable, narrow your scope to the most prevalent denials. The following list provides the areas of focus by the RAC:

- One-day length of stay

- Appropriate place of service and level of care

- Three-day stays

- Medical necessity and setting

- Discharge disposition status codes

- Chest pain

- Congestive heart failure, heart failure and shock

- Medical back pain

- Debridement, especially excisional debridement

- Transfer to inpatient rehabilitation facility (IRF) following joint replacement surgery

- Respiratory system diagnosis with vent support

- Diagnosis designated as complicated or having comorbidity with one secondary Dx

- Extensive OR procedure unrelated to principal diagnosis

- Durable medical equipment items during an inpatient stay

- Colonoscopy

- Speech and language therapy

- Infusion and transfusion services

- High-risk DRGs

- High-volume DRGs

- High-volume outpatient services

- Unit coding

The list is extensive, but using the types of data in your internally developed PEPPER report and comparing it to the above list will provide insight to areas that need continuous monitoring and education on how to properly admit patients.

The areas of opportunities for preventing denials by RACs or any other group is based on the accuracy of documentation for the need for admission. Chapter 1 addresses the CMS definition of medical necessity. Because of the importance of medical necessity in the prevention of RAC denials, it will be further discussed in this chapter. RACs have not provided a definitive method of review. Some have chosen Milliman Care Guidelines, whereas others use InterQual as a guide for determinations. All have stated time and again that their reviews are based on medical necessity as outlined by CMS. The following is the definition provided in the *Medicare Benefit Policy Manual*:

> *An inpatient is a person who has been admitted to a hospital for bed occupancy for purposes of receiving inpatient hospital services. Generally, a patient is considered an inpatient if formally admitted as inpatient with the expectation that he or she will remain at least overnight and occupy a bed, even though it later develops that the patient can be discharged or transferred to another hospital, and not actually use a hospital bed overnight.*

The physician or other practitioner responsible for a patient's care at the hospital is also responsible for deciding whether the patient should be admitted as an inpatient. Physicians should use a 24-hour period as a benchmark, i.e., they should order admission for patients who are expected to need hospital care for 24 hours or more, and treat other patients on an outpatient basis. However, the decision to admit a patient is a complex medical judgment which can be made only after the physician has considered a number of factors, including the patient's medical history and current medical needs, the types of facilities available to inpatients and to outpatients, the hospital's by-laws and admissions policies, and the relative appropriateness of treatment in each setting. Factors to be considered when making the decision to admit include such things as:

- *The severity of the signs and symptoms exhibited by the patient;*

- *The medical predictability of something adverse happening to the patient;*

- *The need for diagnostic studies that appropriately are outpatient services (i.e., their performance does not ordinarily require the patient to remain at the hospital for 24 hours or more) to assist in assessing whether the patient should be admitted; and*

- *The availability of diagnostic procedures at the time when and at the location where the patient presents.*

(Medicare Benefit Policy Manual, Pub 100-02, Rev. 45, 02-10-06).

One key factor in accuracy of documenting the appropriateness of admission is to have the patient's physician include his or her observations about the acuity of the patient's presenting illness, the predictability of an adverse outcome, and a treatment plan that can only be provided at an acute level of care. The reviewers from RAC will be expert utilization nurses and certified coders as outlined in the permanent RAC policies; therefore, the information contained in the medical record needs to be definitive. Ambiguities in medical necessity will most likely result in a denial or require an extended review.

Under the RAC program, the hospital must make a decision to appeal a denial prior to repayment, which can result in interest charges if the appeal is unsuccessful, or pay back the denial and then appeal. Documentation will be key to making the decision to appeal. Involving physicians who understand clinical criteria for determining appropriateness of admission and continued stay in the process of educating other physicians on how to properly document medical necessity is instrumental in denial prevention. All case managers (CM) have dealt with the "social admission" needing a three-day qualifying stay. Medicare's long-standing rule that a patient be on the census for three consecutive midnights to meet medical necessity for the Extended Care Benefit that includes a skilled nursing stay has led to many questionable admissions. As one physician put it, the "pop drop" admission, in which the family can no longer care for its elderly father or mother, has become a prevalent feature of the American healthcare scene. Physicians and hospitals, particularly CMs, are placed in a position of determining how to care for these individuals—truly a social issue. But be aware that, many times, these patients do meet medical necessity. What leads to the denial is not the social status of the admission, but the lack of documentation to demonstrate that the patient cannot be discharged and requires acute care to determine his or her functionality and level of care. CMs argue about this kind of case all of the time. The following case study is a typical example.

CASE STUDY

A 78-year-old female is brought to the ED by her daughter, who states that her mother has had frequent falls, which have increased in the past week with progressive mental deterioration and forgetfulness. The daughter works full time, and there is no one to take care of her mother during the day. She is afraid that her mother will fall and hurt herself if left alone and requests placement into a nursing home. A review of systems reveals a primarily healthy person with some bruising on her knees and elbows from frequent falls. Neurologically, there is short-term memory loss and an inability to maintain focus. Vital signs and labs are within normal limits, except the patient's glucose, which is 297; EKG shows ST-T wave changes of undetermined age. CT of the head reveals age-specific changes with no gross abnormalities. X-rays of the patient's elbow and knees are negative. PMH determines that the patient has HTN, diabetes, and COPD. Her medications include Norvasc, ASA, Atrovent inhaler b.i.d., and Lantus pen q-day with b.i.d. finger sticks.

None of the presenting information indicates a need for acute care. However, if the patient is sent home with proper care, the argument can be stated that the predictability of an adverse outcome increases exponentially, especially if she does not have the ability to monitor her glucose and mental capacity to take her medications. The patient will decompensate rather quickly. It is not the responsibility of healthcare to pass judgment on the daughter's inability to provide further care for her mother, but to find a solution to provide appropriate care. Remember the Medicare definition of an inpatient, which includes: "the decision to admit a patient is a complex medical judgment which can be made only after the physician has considered a number of factors, including the patient's medical history and current medical needs, the types of facilities available to inpatients and to outpatients..."

The definition continues, "Factors to be considered when making the decision to admit include such things as:

- The severity of the signs and symptoms exhibited by the patient
- The medical predictability of something adverse happening to the patient"

In accordance with these factors, the physician should document that discharging the patient home can and most likely will lead to uncontrolled hypertension that can result in stroke, uncontrolled diabetes

---

that can lead to DKA or diabetic coma, and the possibility of a respiratory decompensation that can lead to respiratory arrest as a result of an inability for self-care due to the decreasing mental deterioration as evidenced by an increase in short-term memory loss and declining motor function as evidenced by an increase in frequent falls. The picture painted is very different than the typical history and physical. It is incumbent upon case management and utilization review departments to educate physicians to document in a manner that describes the potential negative impact on the patient if she is not admitted. Admitting orders should then be based on diagnosis, stabilization, and treatment for her neurological problems and physical debilitation that requires physical therapy, neurology consults, MRI, and other steps to determine her new baseline.

InterQual and Milliman are guidelines that insurance companies use as a tool to base the denial of a patient's admission or continued stay for which the hospital submits a claim. Medicare uses these same guidelines to formulate its medical necessity definition but it also incorporates the view that admission and continued stay is based on the physician's judgment and his or her ability to document the needs of the patient.

Review Process and Appeal Process for RAC

The RAC program has timelines that must be adhered to by each party. There are requirements for requesting documents, informing facilities of determinations, providing time to decide an appeal, and the various steps of appeal. The entire timeline for the review process can be lengthy. The following is from the CMS Manual, Pub 100-20, *Transmittal 314*, from July 2008, which discusses recoupment time frames for RACs, but also includes the time frames surrounding each appeal level:

> In addition, to the extent it is feasible and cost-effective to do so, certain new or revised overpayment recovery processes required to fully implement the limitation

on recoupment should be automated. For planning and system design purposes, these changes should reflect the following approach. For Part A overpayments subject to 1893(f)(2), receipt of a timely and valid request for appeal (the contractor redetermination) triggers the limitation on recoupment. Once the contractor has determined the overpayment and adjusted the claim in the Fiscal Intermediary Standard System FISS the withholding of the overpayment will automatically be set to begin withholding 30 days from the determination date. When that day is current, the withholding shall begin if the provider has not submitted an appeal for redetermination (first level of appeal). If an appeal was submitted by the provider within those 30 days, the withholding will not begin. If the contractor redetermination results in a full or partial affirmation of the overpayment, contractors can begin or resume recoupment starting 60 days and no later than 75 days after giving notice unless the provider appeals to the Qualified Independent Contractor (QIC) in the interim. The contractor should cease *or not begin recoupment if the QIC notifies the contractor that a valid and timely request for reconsideration (second level of appeal) has been received. Following final action by the QIC, the contractor can initiate or resume recoupment whether or not the provider subsequently appeals to the administrative law judge (ALJ) (third level of appeal). For a period of up to 60 days following final action by the QIC and resumption of recoupment, Medicare contractors should not issue a second demand letter, the intent to refer letter, nor proceed with referral to the Department of Treasury. Interest will continue to accrue under current policies but will not be assessed when recoupment is stopped at either the redetermination or reconsideration (first and second level of appeals).*

Each denial should be carefully considered. A determination as to whether to proceed with an appeal should be a joint decision between the appeal personnel and the medical and finance staff. The decision to appeal has a significant financial effect:

- The hospital may need to pay interest on the denied amount if the denial is upheld and,

- If the appeal cases proceed to the ALJ level, this will require the assistance of legal counsel to navigate the system.

Money is better spent in preventing the denial by adding additional personnel if needed to reach 100% review for all Medicare admissions. Medicaid has begun to follow suit, and many states now have a similar process to the RAC for recoupment of overpayments. Medicaid claims should not be set aside and should receive the same scrutiny as the Medicare claims.

The flow diagram in **Figure 8.1** suggests a method by which to handle the RAC process and shows the timelines for each step of the process.

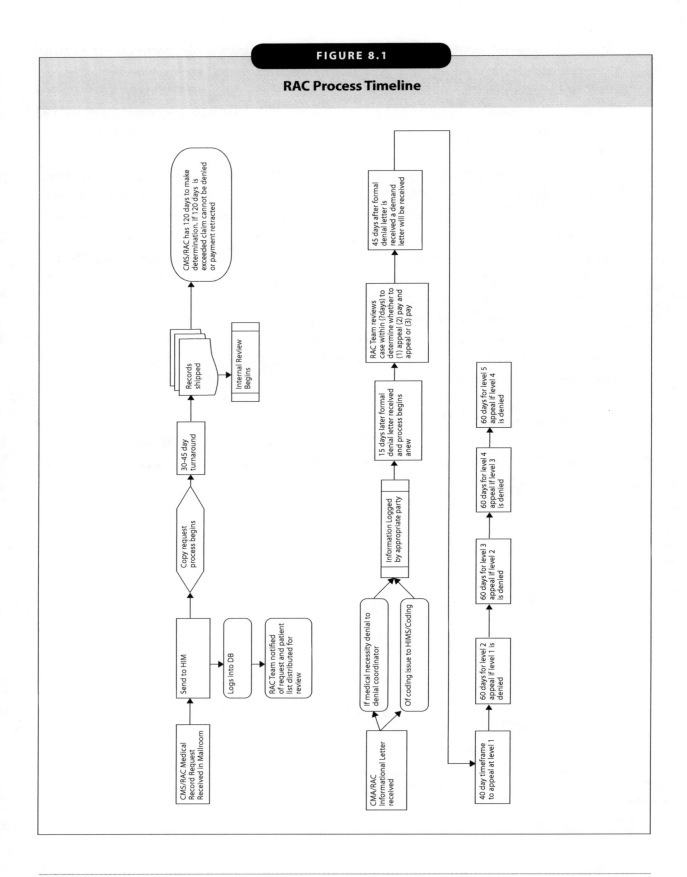

FIGURE 8.1

RAC Process Timeline

Prevent Denials and Win Appeals

Summary

The RAC process has been a whirlwind across the entire U.S. healthcare industry. The final reversal numbers are still not available, but preliminary figures demonstrate that proper documentation will lead to a reversal up to an astounding 100% of the time. Education of the medical staff about how to properly document the need for an acute care stay regardless of the DRG will enable hospitals to overturn frivolous denials. As the RAC denial and appeal process evolves over time, there will be best practice patterns that will help case management staff members to better understand their role and how to assist in the prevention of the RAC denials. A strong point-of-entry review process, including reviewing an admission of a patient through the emergency department, a direct admit, or an admit from observation service, can capture the majority of the high-risk MS-DRGs will help prevent denials and win appeals. Concentration of resources should be used to review the high-risk cases on a daily basis. Tracking denials and creating a PEPPER-like report (see Chapter 7) will ensure that your facility stays ahead of the contractors.

Staying Ahead of the Game

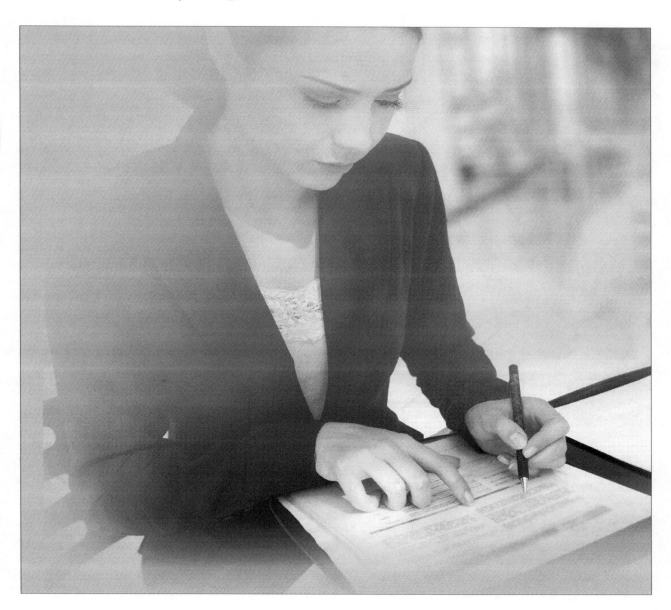

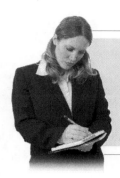

Staying Ahead of the Game

CHAPTER 9

Being Alert to the Issues

Laws, regulations, mandates, accrediting bodies, and other entities have an effect on denials and appeals. Chapter 1 began with an overview of the history of medical necessity and discussed the various regulations that have been created over time to reach the current state of healthcare. The Social Security Act of 1965 established Medicare and Medicaid. Since that time, regulations on how to provide coverage have expanded to the point where, as of October 2008, hospitals are no longer reimbursed at a higher MS-DRG if certain conditions are present on admission, which means a complication was acquired during a hospital stay, or if a never event, such as wrong-site surgery, occurs. Other aspects of the Social Security Act under Title XVIII established guidelines for the creation of utilization review (UR) and discharge planning. The federal government creates laws and subsequently provides regulations that enforce the laws. Proposed regulations are published in the *Federal Register*. During the enactment of a new or a changing regulation, there are open comment periods during which opinions are solicited from experts in the field to help determine what effect regulations will have. There may be some question about how rules and regulations are proposed and passed or about many of the government's healthcare decisions, but the system in this country allows

LEARNING OBJECTIVES

At the end of the chapter, the reader should be able to:

- ✔ Identify where and how to find changes to regulations

- ✔ Describe the regulations that govern medical necessity

- ✔ Track potential changes to healthcare that may impact case management and utilization review

everyone to participate and be heard during the comment period. It is remarkable that so few of us make comments when our views can make a difference.

Case management should be an active participant in issues that affect patient care. It is incumbent upon us to be advocates for patients and for our employers. Case management associations such as the American Case Management Association (ACMA) and the Case Management Society of America (CMSA) are active participants in lobbying efforts as advocates for the healthcare industry. One method of maintaining the pulse of changes is by being actively involved in these and other associations that partake in lobbying Congress on behalf of patients. Listservs, blogs, weekly e-mail alerts, and monthly journals are other rich sources of information. A proactive case management staff can help lead to successes, such as being able to discern significant changes and act accordingly. The states that participated in the RAC demonstration project gained valuable information and are now considered experts on how to deal with RAC denials. They developed tools and best practices that have enabled them to protect and defend potential and actual denials. Knowing where to look and how to screen for information is a skill that needs honing and can take time to master, but it is not the proverbial rocket science. It requires reading, discussion, and the ability to set up automatic e-mails and participate in discussion groups. The ACMA has an extremely active listserv on which members can pose questions and receive relevant answers. HCPro, Inc., recently launched a case management blog that also has relevant information, including commentary from experts in the field.

How to Find Regulation Changes and Incorporate Them into the Appeals Process

To be effective in any appeals process, you must understand the regulations and laws that affect the ability to obtain information. Additionally, being able to accurately quote applicable rules and regulations adds authority to your argument to receive reimbursement for the services provided. Rules, laws, and regulations have been challenged in many ways that often require our court system to make

determinations about the meaning and intent of the lawmakers. Hospitals, patients, consumer advocates, and insurance companies have availed themselves of legal proceedings to determine who is right and wrong, or simply to decide the meaning of wording. However, each decision made by the courts can set a precedent, especially at the U.S. Court of Appeals or Supreme Court level, or even at the highest court in each state. It is not necessary to become lawyers or hang out in courts, but to better understand the ramifications of court decisions, you must be aware of the judicial decisions that affect the interpretation of laws and regulations. The world of information technology available to us today is unprecedented in its ability to retrieve information instantly. Most search engines provide relevant search terms and will display an array of useful information. Entering the terms "medical necessity" and "Supreme Court" into the most common search engine, Google™, yields more than 600,000 hits. Of course, that is too many returns to read, but the idea is that by using common search terms, you can retrieve information that is relevant to your field. For example, one such search result through Google is the 2003 case of *Aetna v. Davila* in which the Supreme Court ruled that in cases of interpretation of a beneficiary's plan that affects the duty to pay (fiduciary duty), federal rules (ERISA) totally preempt state laws. The effect of that case was felt by the insurance companies that hid behind state laws that at times were not friendly to beneficiaries. It also opened the doors to use ERISA in ways that were previously protected by state laws, in which a hospital could not rely on the federal laws to obtain information such as who made the denial determination, what documents were used for the determination, and even to force the insurance company to provide the denial in a letter format with the denial reason, the appeal process, and the timeline for appeals. Many denials are sent to hospitals on the explanation of benefits as a line-item denial. If the beneficiary has a plan that was purchased through his employer, he is covered under ERISA and thus entitled to the full protection of the regulation requiring the insurance company to provide a full disclosure of the denial and the appeals process through the assignment of rights to the hospital.

Access to laws, regulations, and determinations is free in most states and also free from the federal government. Some insurance companies, through the provision of provider agreements, may charge a nominal per page fee to reproduce documents.

The CMS Web site, *www.cms.hhs.gov*, has a wealth of information but can be tricky to navigate. Using precise terms and Boolean operators in the site's search engine will help you get the information you need.

Most states have their own Web sites to help users access laws. Spend some time navigating these sites to access the public health laws and insurance laws that affect your ability to appeal denials and learn how to access insurance review agents in cases in which a dispute cannot be resolved in the first two levels of appeals. Many state insurance agencies will review only retrospective denials, thus removing themselves from the decision-making process that may affect current treatment options.

Other useful Web sites on which regulations and interpretations to processes may be found are states' quality improvement organization (QIO) sites. Each state has a QIO that is dedicated to review of Medicare and Medicaid cases. Hospitals should have a designated liaison who interacts with the QIO to create a working relationship that will be beneficial in understanding its processes and who to go to for information. In New York, the author worked closely with the Island Professional Review Organization (IPRO), which has the federal and state contract for Medicare and Medicaid. IPRO maintains a Web site that is dedicated to patients, providers, and professionals. It also provides seminars and live contacts to answer questions, as well as educational forums and letters. Most state QIOs do the same. When the Important Message from Medicare (needed to provide appeals rights to Medicare beneficiaries) was launched, the QIOs were responsible for the administration of the appeals and denial process and, as such, were entrusted with providing education on the new regulations.

Private entities are also a rich source of information, such as the Kaiser Foundation, the American Hospital Association, and the AMA, to name a few.

Laws that Govern Medical Necessity

Laws are enacted in the United States at different levels. Our constitution guarantees certain separations between federal and state governments. What most of us have encountered is that not all laws are separate or easy to interpret and that many overlap, such as the case of ERISA and state laws. Medicare also has regulations, such as national and local determination policies, that affect reimbursement and approval of services, as follows:

National Coverage Determination (NCD). Medicare coverage is limited to items and services that are reasonable and necessary for the diagnosis or treatment of an illness or injury (and within the scope of a Medicare benefit category). The NCDs are developed by CMS to describe the circumstances for which Medicare will cover specific services, procedures, or technologies on a national basis. Medicare contractors are required to follow NCDs. If an NCD does not specifically exclude/limit an indication or circumstance, or if the item or service is not mentioned at all in an NCD or in a Medicare manual, it is up to the Medicare contractor to make the coverage decision.

Local Coverage Determinations (LCD). In the absence of a national coverage policy, an item or service may be covered at the discretion of the Medicare contractors based on a local coverage determination (LCD).

Section 522 of the Benefits Improvement and Protection Act (BIPA) defines an LCD as a decision by a FI or carrier whether to cover a particular service on an intermediary-wide or carrier-wide basis in accordance with Section 1862(a)(1)(A) of the Social Security Act (e.g., a determination as to whether the service or item is reasonable and necessary). (www.cms.hhs.gov/MedicalReviewProcess/)

If there is a doubt about how a law affects your ability to perform your duties, seek clarification from counsel. Lawyers are expensive, but the return on investment can lead to a complete recoupment and a profit on the information. For example, what to do with a patient who has been sent to your facility by a nursing home because the nursing home could not get information on the patient's finances to complete the

Medicaid application and refuses to accept the patient back? The nursing home is not being paid and has no leverage to get the family to comply. Since the patient came out of your facility, the nursing home transfers the long-term care patient back to you and expects you to find a solution. After assessing the patient, you discover there is no medically necessary care that needs to be provided at the acute care setting, and if you do admit the patient, you will not get paid. Most states will not allow the nursing home to "drop" a patient in this manner, as it is considered an eviction from the patient's permanent residence. This is a scenario in which legal counsel can provide you with the information necessary to persuade the nursing home to accept the patient back and follow the legal process of eviction. Knowing how to access and communicate information can lead to a decreased denial rate.

The Future State of Healthcare

Some of the author's recent discussions have centered on the continuum of care model. Patient care is fragmented into episodes of care at different levels without the progression necessary to affect ongoing care, outcomes, and quality. You might be wondering how this relates to denial prevention and appeals. Readmissions, avoidable days, and delays can be attributed to poor-quality discharge planning and inadequate community resources. Hospital case management and UR programs have the data to support the investment in programs that will place patients at the correct level of care at the right time. Many politicians think they have the answers to healthcare, but those in healthcare have firsthand information. Let's dare to dream of an encounter with the senator or congressman from your state in which you present denial and appeal data and can demonstrate how many lives were affected by a proposed readmission rule that denies payment to hospitals if a patient is readmitted within 30 days. If each hospital presented the billions of dollars spent on treating readmissions that occurred due to patient noncompliance, lack of postacute care follow-up, and the inability for a patient to be seen in a timely manner by a private physician, do you think it might be changed? How about care for the congestive heart failure patient, another class of patients on the radar for denials, if we provided a transition of care that included a transition coach and home infusion therapy for repeated exacerbations—how many billions of dollars would be saved? Case management and UR departments have a wealth of information that needs to be quantified and qualified in a collective fashion to present the reasons and solutions to many of our healthcare woes. Companies have started to collect avoidable days/delays data. What if they were shared with our legislatures and demonstrated the amount of unfunded patients who cannot get postacute care and the cost to the acute care system—would we see a paradigm shift in funding? The data that are collected in the denial and appeals process are powerful and need to be harnessed to be effective. Creating a trillion-dollar national healthcare database is not the solution. We have the data; we simply need to share and aggregate them and take action.

The future of denial prevention will be centered on point of access to review cases at admission in collaboration with the medical staff. "Admit by Case Management Protocol" has been viewed as an answer. But recent interpretation from National Government Services stated that, although a protocol can determine the admission status through medical necessity, it is not effective until the physician actually signs the order as evidence of the need for physician and case management collaboration.

Summary

Denial prevention will be an ever-evolving process as long as we maintain our current healthcare system, and those involved will need to be prepared to deal with the changes and access information as needed. Looking ahead, we are likely to see case management placed outside the walls of the hospital and into the community as part of the hospital organization.

Glossary

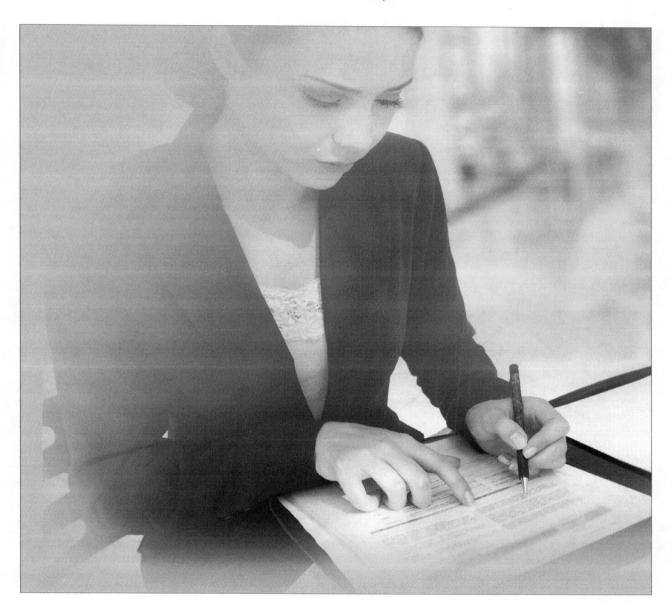

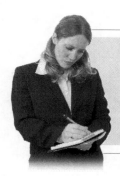

Glossary

The following glossary is from the CMS Manual System, Pub 100-04 Medicare Claims Processing (Rev. 1762, Issued: 07-02-09, Effective: 08-03-09, Implementation: 08-03-09).

Adjudicator

The entity responsible for making the decision at any level of the Medicare claim decision making process, from initial determination to the final level of appeal on a specific claim.

Administrative Law Judge (ALJ)

Adjudicator employed by the U.S. Department of Health and Human Services, Office of Medicare Hearings and Appeals.

Affirmation

A term used to denote that a prior claims determination has been upheld by the current claims adjudicator. Although appeals through the ALJ level are de novo, CMS and its contractors often use this term when a reviewer reaches the same conclusion as that in the prior determination, even though he/she is not bound by the prior determination.

Amount in Controversy

The dollar amount required to be in dispute to establish the right to a particular level of appeal. Congress establishes the amount in controversy requirements.

Appellant

The term used to designate the party (i.e., the beneficiary, provider, supplier, or other person showing an interest in the claim determination) or the representative of the party that has filed an appeal. The adjudicator determines if a particular appellant is a proper party or representative of a proper party.

Appointed representative

The individual appointed by a party to represent the party in a Medicare claim or claim appeal.

Assignee

(1) With respect to the assignment of a claim for items or services, the assignee is the supplier who has furnished items or services to a beneficiary and has accepted a valid assignment of a claim OR (2) With respect to an assignment of appeal rights, an assignee is a provider or supplier who is not already a party to an appeal, who has furnished items or services to a beneficiary, and has accepted a valid assignment of the right to appeal a claim executed by the beneficiary.

Assignment of appeal rights

The transfer by a beneficiary of his or her right to appeal under the claims appeal process to a provider or supplier who is not already a party, and who provided the items or services to the beneficiary.

Assignor

A beneficiary whose provider of service or supplier has taken assignment of a claim, or assignment of an appeal of a claim.

Authorized representative

An individual authorized under State or other applicable law to act on behalf of a beneficiary or other party involved in the appeal. The authorized representative will have all of the rights and responsibilities of a beneficiary or party, as applicable, throughout the appeals process.

Beneficiary

Individual who is enrolled to receive benefits under Medicare Part A or Part B.

Departmental Appeals Board (DAB) review

The part of the DAB that reviews Medicare cases is called the Medicare Appeals Council (herein Appeals Council). A party to the ALJ hearing may request review by the Appeals Council within 60 days after receipt of the notice of the ALJ's hearing decision or dismissal. The Appeals Council conducts a de novo review of the ALJ decision, and may adopt, modify or reverse the ALJ's decision, or may remand the case to an ALJ for further proceedings. In reviewing an ALJ's dismissal order, the Appeals Council may deny review or vacate the dismissal and remand the case to an ALJ for further proceedings. The Appeals Council will dismiss a request for review when a party does not have a right to Appeals Council review. The Appeals Council may also dismiss a request for a hearing for any reason the ALJ could have dismissed the request for hearing.

The Appeals Council may also decide on its own motion to review a decision or dismissal issued by an ALJ within 60 days after the date of the hearing decision or dismissal. In addition, CMS may refer a case to the Appeals Council for it to consider under its own motion review authority within 60 days after the date of the hearing decision or dismissal. This is known as an "Agency Referral". The Appeals Council may adopt, modify, or reverse the ALJ's decision, may remand the case to an ALJ for further proceedings, or may dismiss an Agency Referral request.

De novo

Latin phrase meaning "anew" or "afresh," used to denote the manner in which claims are adjudicated through the ALJ level of appeal. Adjudicators at each level of appeal make a new, independent and thorough evaluation of the claim(s) at issue, and are not bound by the findings and decision made by an adjudicator in a prior determination or decision.

Decisions and determinations

If a Medicare appeal request does not result in a dismissal, adjudication of the appeal results in either a "determination" or "decision." There is no apparent practical distinction between these two terms although applicable regulations use the terms in distinct contexts.

A decision that is reopened and thereafter revised is called a "revised determination."

Dismissal

- A request for appeal may be dismissed for any number of reasons, including:

- Abandonment of the appeal by the appellant;

- A request is made by the appellant to withdraw the appeal;

- An appellant is determined to not be a proper party;

- The amount in controversy requirements have not been met; and

- The appellant has died and no one else is prejudiced by the claims determination.

Parties to the redetermination have the right to appeal a dismissal of a redetermination request to a qualified independent contractor (QIC) if they believe the dismissal is incorrect. If the QIC determines that the contractor incorrectly dismissed the redetermination, it will vacate the dismissal and remand the case to the contractor for a redetermination. It is mandatory for the contractor to conduct a redetermination on any case that is remanded to it by the QIC and issue a new decision. A QIC's decision upon reconsideration of a contractor's dismissal of a redetermination request, including a QIC's dismissal of the reconsideration request if untimely filed, is binding and not subject to further review.

Limitation on liability determination

Section 1879 of the Social Security Act (the Act) provides financial relief to beneficiaries, providers and suppliers by permitting Medicare payment to be made, or requiring refunds to be made, for certain services and items for which Medicare coverage and payment would otherwise be denied. This section of the Act is referred to as "the limitation on liability provision." Both the underlying coverage determination and the limitation on liability determination may be challenged.

Party

A person and/or entity normally understood to have standing to appeal an initial determination and/or a subsequent administrative appeal determination or decision. Parties to the initial determination include:

- Beneficiaries, who are almost always considered parties to a Medicare determination, as they are entitled to appeal any initial determination (unless the beneficiary has assigned his or her appeal rights).

- Providers who file a claim for items or services furnished to a beneficiary.

- Participating suppliers.

Parties to the redetermination and subsequent appeal levels include:

- The parties to the initial determination, above

- Non-participating suppliers accepting assignment of a claim for items or services (but only for the items or services which they have billed on an assigned basis).

- A non-participating physician not billing on an assigned basis but who may be responsible for making a refund to the beneficiary under §1842(l)(1) of the Act for services furnished to a beneficiary that are denied on the basis of section 1862(a)(1) of the Act, has party status with respect to the claim at issue.

- A non-participating supplier not billing on an assigned basis, who may be responsible for making a refund to the beneficiary under §1834(a)(18) or §1834(j)(4) of the Act has party status with respect to the claim at issue.

- Medicaid State agencies have party status at the redetermination level (and subsequent levels) for claims for items or services involving a beneficiary who is enrolled to receive benefits under both Medicare and Medicaid, but only if the Medicaid state agency has made payment for, or may be liable for such items or services, and only if the State agency has filed a timely request for redetermination for such items or services. See 42 CFR 405.908.

- A provider or supplier who has furnished items or services to a beneficiary that |does not otherwise have appeal rights, but has accepted an assignment of appeal rights from the beneficiary pursuant to 42 CFR 405.912 (but only with respect to the claims identified in the assignment agreement).

Provider of services (herein provider)

As used in this section, the definition in 42 *CFR* 405.902 for provider applies. Provider means a hospital, a critical access hospital (CAH), a skilled nursing facility, a comprehensive outpatient rehabilitation facility, a home health agency, or a hospice that has in effect an agreement to participate in Medicare, or a clinic, a rehabilitation agency, or a public health agency that has in effect a similar agreement but only to furnish outpatient physical therapy or speech pathology services, or a community mental health center that has in effect a similar agreement but only to furnish partial hospitalization services.

Qualified independent contractor (QIC)

An entity that contracts with the Secretary in accordance with the Act to perform reconsiderations and expedited reconsiderations.

Remand

An action taken by an adjudicator to vacate a lower level appeal decision, or a portion of the decision, and return the case, or a portion of the case, to that level for a new decision.

Reversal

Although appeals through the ALJ hearing level are de novo proceedings (i.e., a new determination/decision is made at each level), Medicare uses this term where the new determination/decision is more favorable to the appellant than the prior determination/decision, even if some aspects of the prior determination/decision remain the same.

Note: the term reversal describes the coverage determination, not the liability determination. For example, an item or service may be determined to be non-covered as not medically reasonable and necessary (under section 1862(a)(1)(A) of the Act), but Medicare may, nevertheless, make payment for the item or service if the party is found not financially liable after applying the limitation on liability provision (section 1879 of the Act). Thus, the coverage determination is affirmed, but Medicare makes payment as required by statute.

Revised determination or decision

An initial determination or decision that is reopened and which results in the issuance of a revised determination or decision. A revised determination or decision is considered a separate and distinct determination or decision and may be appealed. For example, a post-payment review of an initial determination that results in a reversal of a previously covered/paid claim (and, potentially, a subsequent overpayment determination) constitutes a reopening and a revised initial determination. The first level of appeal following a revised initial determination is a redetermination.

Supplier

A supplier includes a physician or other practitioner, a facility, or other entity (other than a provider of services) that furnishes items or services under Medicare. Unless the context otherwise requires, a physician or other practitioner, a facility, or entity (other than a provider) that furnishes items or services under Medicare.

Vacate

To set aside a previous action.

CMS Resources

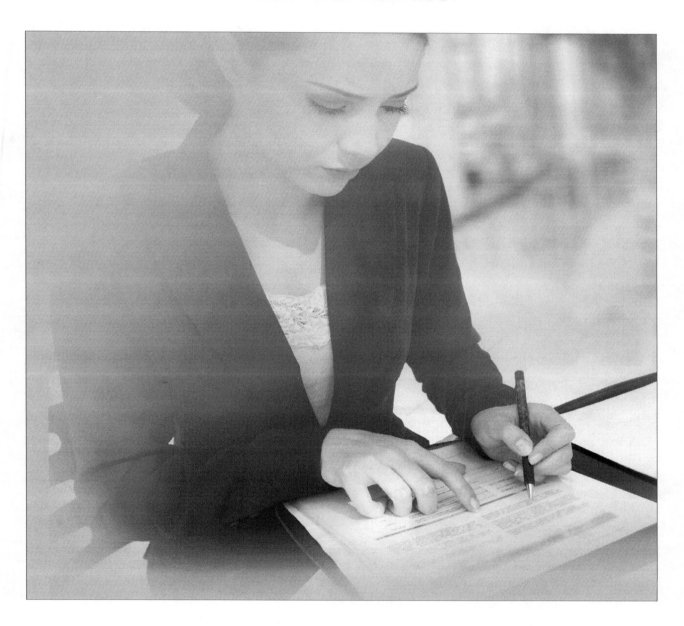

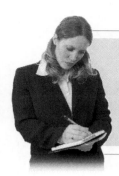

CMS Resources

Here is a list of helpful resources on the CMS Web site, which are also included on the CD-ROM.

1. Medicare *Claims Processing Manual*, Chapters 3, 4: *www.cms.hhs.gov/Manuals/IOM/itemdetail. asp?filterType=none&filterByDID=-99&sortByDID=1&sortOrder=ascending&itemID=CMS018912*

2. Transmittal 1745 - Medicare Claims Processing: *www.cms.hhs.gov/Transmittals/Downloads/ R1745CP.pdf*

3. Chapter IV - Centers for Medicare & Medicaid Services, Department of Health and Human Services (continued) PART 482--Conditions of Participation for Hospitals – UR and D/C Planning: *www.access. gpo.gov/nara/cfr/waisidx_05/42cfr482_05.html*

4. Employee Retirement Income Security Act of 1974; Rules and Regulations for Administration and Enforcement; Claims Procedure; Final Rule [11/21/2000] - Volume 65, Number 225, Page 70245- 70271: *www.dol.gov/ebsa/regs/fedreg/final/2000029766.htm*

5. National Determination Coverage Policies: *www.cms.hhs.gov/Manuals/IOM/itemdetail. asp?filterType=none&filterByDID=-99&sortByDID=1&sortOrder=ascending&itemID=CMS014961*

6. Appeals Revision: *www.cms.hhs.gov/transmittals/downloads/R1762CP.pdf*

7. RAC Transmittal 152: *www.cms.hhs.gov/Transmittals/Downloads/R152FM. pdf*

8. *State Operations Manual* Appendix A - Regulations and Interpretive Guidelines for Hospitals: *www.cms.hhs.gov/manuals/downloads/som107ap_a_hospitals.pdf*

Instructional Guide

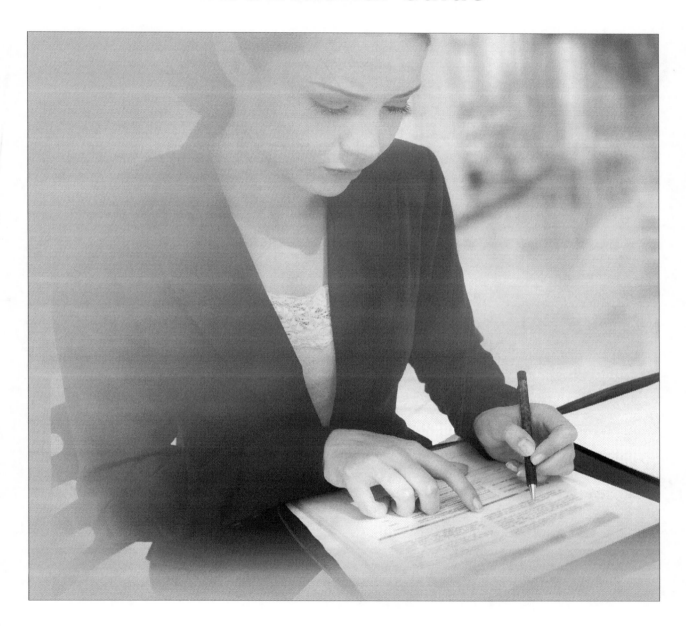

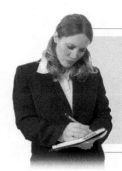

Target Audience

- Directors of case management

- Hospital case managers

Statement of Need

As federal and private payers look to reduce costs, they are taking a closer look at medical necessity and utilization review. This book will show case managers how to also prevent appeals on the front end by managing level of care decisions, identifying cost/revenue, distilling payer methodology and contract language, and zeroing in on proper documentation practices. It will also instruct hospitals on how to track and trend denials to understand their root cause and implement prevention strategies to create an airtight retrospective appeal process. Above all, this book will show readers how to identify the issues and trends at their organization and how to understand and pinpoint whether their denials are payer issues or internal issues.

Educational Objectives

Upon completion of this activity, participants should be able to:

- Define the basis of medical necessity.

- Explain how the case management function fits within the prevention of denials.

- Define utilization review (UR).

- Identify sources of evidence-based medicine.

- Relate how criteria guidelines are derived.

- Define denial prevention.

- State the role of the physician advisor in terms of denial prevention.

- Identify strategies to track denial prevention.

- Discuss where case management and denial prevention fit within the revenue cycle.

- Describe ways to partner with the finance department.

- Calculate the savings and offset the losses of denials.

- Describe the appeals process.

- Identify steps to ensure a high reversal rate.

- Identify what data to report.

- Determine how to best organize the data.

- Determine to whom the data should be reported.

- Define the relationship between contracting and denial prevention.

- Articulate language that should be included in contracts with payers to ensure compliance with regulations.

- Understand the genesis of RAC.

- Implement strategies to prevent RAC denials.

- Identify location and how to find changes to regulations.

- Understand the law that governs medical necessity.

Faculty

Paul Arias, RN, BSN, MIS, is the senior director of case management at Inova Fairfax Hospital in Falls Church, VA. He was most recently the director of care coordination at Crouse Hospital in Syracuse, NY, which maintained a denial rate of less than 1% and a 72% reversal rate under his leadership. In more than 14 years as a nurse, Arias has been primarily in leadership roles, including ED manager, critical care director, and chief executive nurse/director of patient care services. He was a copresenter for HCPro's audio conference, "Prevent Denials Through Case Management."

Nursing Contact Hours

HCPro, Inc., is accredited as a provider of continuing nursing education by the American Nurses Credentialing Center Commission on Accreditation. This educational activity for 3 nursing contact hours is provided by HCPro, Inc.

Commission for Case Manager Certification (CCMC)

This activity has been approved by the Commission for Case Manager Certification for 6 Continuing Education Units.

Disclosure Statements

HCPro, Inc., has confirmed that none of the faculty or contributors have any relevant financial relationships to disclose related to the content of this educational activity.

Instructions

To be eligible to receive your nursing contact hours or case manager continuing education credits for this activity, you are required to do the following:

1. Read *Prevent Denials and Win Appeals*.

2. Complete the exam and receive a passing score of 80%.

3. Complete the evaluation.

4. Provide your contact information on the exam and evaluation.

5. Submit the exam and evaluation to HCPro, Inc.

Please provide all of the information requested above and mail or fax your completed exam, program evaluation, and contact information to:

HCPro, Inc.
Attn: Continuing Education Manager
P.O. Box 1168
Marblehead, MA 01945
Fax: 781/639-2982

NOTE:

This book and associated exam are intended for individual use only. If you would like to provide this continuing education exam to other members of your nursing or physician staff, please contact our customer service department at 877/727-1728 to place your order. The exam fee schedule is as follows:

Exam quantity	Fee
1	$0
2–25	$15 per person
26–50	$12 per person
51–100	$8 per person
101+	$5 per person

CONTINUING EDUCATION EXAM

Name: _____

Title: _____

Facility name: _____

Address: _____

Address: _____

City: _____ State: _____ ZIP: _____

Phone number: _____ Fax number: _____

E-mail: _____

Date completed: _____

1. **Medical necessity was established by Medicare as means to provide cost-effective care and to:**
   a. Limit the physician in indiscriminately requesting admission or continued stay
   b. Allow the physician greater flexibility in requesting admission or continued stay
   c. Limit the physician's role in determining the patient's length of stay (LOS)
   d. Ensure that the physician is the sole decision-maker of the patient's admission status

2. **The ED case manager helps with denial prevention by:**
   a. Monitoring patients who are frequently admitted to the ED and may be "frequent flyers"
   b. Assisting the physician in identifying patients who do not meet acute care admission criteria
   c. Assessing patients for postdischarge needs prior to inpatient admission
   d. All of the above

3. **What are the two most prevalently used criteria for utilization review (UR)?**
   a. InterQual and Milliman Care Guidelines
   b. InterQual and PubMed
   c. Milliman Care Guidelines and Google™
   d. Milliman and PubMed

4. **What is the primary driver behind the creation of criteria guidelines?**
   a. The hospital's administration team
   b. CINHAL
   c. Evidence-based medicine
   d. None of the above

5. **Denial prevention begins when:**
   a. The patient enters the system
   b. The patient is admitted to acute care
   c. The case manager sees the patient
   d. The physician sees the patient

6. **Which of the following can a physician advisor do as an integral part of the case management (CM) department?**
   a. Bridge the gap to the medical staff
   b. Provide support for review
   c. Act as co-chair for the UR committee
   d. All of the above

7. **How often should patient data be reviewed for denial trends?**
   a. At least once per year
   b. At least twice per year
   c. At least once per month
   d. Every week

8. **How can case management have a positive effect on the revenue cycle?**
   a. Through UR
   b. Decreasing LOS
   c. Issuing denial letters
   d. All of the above

9. **The data that are presented to any chief officer should be delivered in a manner that will:**
   a. Encourage questioning about the data
   b. Prevent questioning of the data's validity
   c. Require time and scrutiny to interpret
   d. Show information from only a one-week timeline

10. **Trends should be correlated with any denials that affect payment:**
    a. At the front end of the stay
    b. At the back end of the stay
    c. In the middle of the stay
    d. At any point during the stay

11. **Which of the following about writing appeal letters is *NOT* true?**
    a. The letter should be addressed to the individual or agent who will determine the outcome of the case.
    b. All appeal letters should be structured in a manner that is consistent with presenting facts to a physician.
    c. The body of the letter should end with a recap of the denial.
    d. Cookie-cutter templates are not effective.

12. **Which of the following is the foundation that must be in place to ensure a high reversal rate?**
    a. Staff education on how to write denial letters
    b. Staff education on how to properly perform reviews
    c. Training of front-end staff members to screen patients
    d. Tracking database for anecdotal evidence

13. **In identifying which data to report, what is the first step?**
    a. Understanding how denials occur
    b. Asking your manager what to report
    c. Creating a database
    d. Meeting with the finance team

14. **Who should receive the denials report?**
    a. Only the physician and the nurses
    b. Only the physician and case managers
    c. The hospital CEO and CFO
    d. All personnel who make admission status decisions

15. **Contracts or agreements between a hospital and a private insurance company are primarily designed to provide a reimbursement methodology that is:**
    a. Beneficial to both parties
    b. Beneficial primarily to the hospital
    c. Beneficial primarily to the patient
    d. Intended to maximize the patient's benefits

16. **Which of the following statements is false regarding contract language?**
    a. Agreements contain language on how the review process is conducted and who will conduct it.
    b. Most case management departments do not get involved in prehospital reviews.
    c. Regulations that affect the dispute resolution process must be included in the agreement.
    d. The areas that most affect case management are the concurrent and restrospective review processes.

17. **The RAC program is expected to investigate claims from as far back as:**
    a. October 2005
    b. October 2006
    c. October 2007
    d. October 2008

18. **The complex review method used by RAC is:**
    a. An automatic screening of the claim for payment errors
    b. A review of the medical records by a team of physicians
    c. A review of the medical record by a claim reviewer
    d. None of these
    e.

19. **Which of the following statements is false?**
    a. Each state has a QIO that is dedicated to review of Medicare and Medicaid cases.
    b. Most states have their own Web sites that help users access laws.
    c. Proposed regulations to existing laws are published in the *Federal Register*.
    d. Regulations and mandates have little effect on denials and appeals.

20. **If an item or service is not mentioned in an NCD or Medicare manual, who makes the coverage decision?**
    a. Medicare contractor
    b. Treating physician
    c. Local government
    d. None of the above

CONTINUING EDUCATION EXAM ANSWER KEY

Please record the letter of the correct answer to the corresponding exam question below:				
1.	5.	9.	13.	17.
2.	6.	10.	14.	18.
3.	7.	11.	15.	19.
4.	8.	12.	16.	20.

Continuing Education Evaluation:

1= Strongly Agree	2 = Agree	3= Disagree	4= Strongly Disagree

(Please rate the responses below according to the scale above to rate the quality of this educational activity)

1. **Please indicate how well you feel this activity met the learning objectives listed:**
   ❏ 1   ❏ 2   ❏ 3   ❏ 4

2. **Objectives were related to the overall purpose/goal of the activity:**
   ❏ 1   ❏ 2   ❏ 3   ❏ 4

3. **This activity was related to my continuing education needs:**
   ❏ 1   ❏ 2   ❏ 3   ❏ 4

4. **The exam for the activity was an accurate test of the knowledge gained:**
   ❏ 1   ❏ 2   ❏ 3   ❏ 4

5. **The activity avoided commercial bias or influence:**
   ❏ 1   ❏ 2   ❏ 3   ❏ 4

6. **This activity met my expectations:**
   ❏ 1   ❏ 2   ❏ 3   ❏ 4

7. **The format was an appropriate method for delivery of the content for this activity:**
   ❏ 1   ❏ 2   ❏ 3   ❏ 4

8. **Will this activity enhance your professional practice?**
   ❏ Yes   ❏ No

9. How much time did it take for you to complete this activity?

_____

10. Do you have any additional comments on this activity?

_____

_____

_____

_____

Return completed form to:

HCPro, Inc.
Attn: Continuing Education Manager
PO Box 1168,
Marblehead, MA 01945

Tel 877/727-1728 • Fax 781/639-2982

FREE HEALTHCARE COMPLIANCE AND MANAGEMENT RESOURCES!

Need to control expenses yet stay current with critical issues?

Get timely help with FREE e-mail newsletters from HCPro, Inc., the leader in healthcare compliance education. Offering numerous free electronic publications covering a wide variety of essential topics, you'll find just the right e-newsletter to help you stay current, informed, and effective. All you have to do is sign up!

With your FREE subscriptions, you'll also receive the following:

- Timely information, to be read when convenient with your schedule
- Expert analysis you can count on
- Focused and relevant commentary
- Tips to make your daily tasks easier

And here's the best part—there's no further obligation—just a complimentary resource to help you get through your daily challenges.

It's easy. Visit *www.hcmarketplace.com/free/e-newsletters/* to register for as many free e-newsletters as you'd like, and let us do the rest.

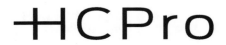
HCPro | Insight for healthcare compliance and management